The Busy Woman's Guide to Losing Weight and Making Money

Karen Fernandez

BALBOA.
PRESS
A DIVISION OF HAY HOUSE

Balboa Press books may be ordered through booksellers or by contacting:

Balboa Press
A Division of Hay House
1663 Liberty Drive
Bloomington, IN 47403
www.balboapress.com.au
1-(877) 407-4847

ISBN: 978-1-4525-0936-5 (sc)
ISBN: 978-1-4525-0937-2 (e)

Printed in the United States of America

Balboa Press rev. date: 03/28/2013

Contents

About the Author

Karen Fernandez was born in Malaysia and migrated to Australia with her parents in 1978. Her family initially lived in small towns in country New South Wales, before finally settling in Sydney. Karen enjoyed writing and art, while she was growing up and dreamed of one day writing her own novel. She spent her high school years in Sydney and went to the University of Wollongong in Wollongong; she completed a Bachelor of Commerce majoring in Accounting.

After completing her degree, Karen secured a Graduate Traineeship at the Office of State Revenue in New South Wales. She worked in the Department for a few years, then moved to Melbourne and got married. While raising her three children she worked in a variety of accounting roles. Karen was always interested in real estate and in 2001 she started to invest in property. In 2004 she divorced and now lives with her children in Melbourne. She currently works full time as an accountant and a meditation teacher.

It is important to Karen that women believe in themselves. She is also a motivational coach who has a passion to help women achieve their goals. Karen inspires others to believe in themselves so that they can have more positive relationships, achieve weight loss and have a better understanding of money.

Karen has written a book to encourage women to make positive changes to their relationships, weight and finances. Her book was born from a genuine desire to help women find happiness in their life, regardless of their past.

She continues to balance her work as an accountant, meditation teacher, property investor, coach and writer while raising her children. She loves to read, watch movies, draw and paint and sculpt clay to relax.

Karen's perfect idea of a relaxing day would be to lie beside a pool (in the shade) with a good book.

Introduction

Whenever women feel bad and are stressed, they either eat or go shopping. We all have those days where something has happened at work or at home so we devour a block of chocolate or buy that dress to make ourselves feel better. It only becomes a problem if we notice that we have weight issues or money problems or both. This is a sign that we are in pain and need to start making changes in our lives and taking better care of ourselves. This situation is complicated because we need to eat daily and spend money in order to live. Therefore we tread a delicate tightrope. Our relationships with people, food, money, and more importantly ourselves are something we need to understand so that our lives are better.

I had my wakeup call when I got divorced and found that I was struggling with every area of my life, in particular my relationships, weight and money. When I got married I had thought it was for life, so when I became separated from my husband, it was totally unexpected. No one had ever talked to me about divorce. Cinderella met her Prince, got married and lived happily ever after. There was no fairy tale about Cinderella getting divorced from her Prince and seeing a lawyer, so that they could divide their assets and make custody arrangements for their children. The reality of my divorce hit me hard and I struggled as I tried to come to terms with the changes in my life. It was the lowest point in my life and I began to question everything. Surely life was not meant to be so difficult.

I started to wonder why I seemed to be attracting the same type of relationships. Why I had issues with losing weight and keeping it off. Why I was suddenly struggling with money. Surely I could lead a life where I had loving and supportive relationships, be my perfect weight and have plenty of money for me and my children. I started reading and searching for answers, and then one day two friends recommended that I read the same book. I am never one to ignore 'signs', so I read the book and it was as though a light had been switched on in my life.

The book talked about how we attracted everything into our lives. I am an accountant by profession so I was a bit sceptical in the beginning. Initially I did my own research, analysed my own life and read a wide range of books. I also started to experiment with strategies in my own life and found the ones that actually worked.

My life started to change and I am now surrounded by loving, supportive relationships. I am my perfect weight and have plenty of money to support me and my children. If I can do it, then so can you. So I have written a book that shows you how to use the strategies to improve your life.

I am a working mum with children, so I know how precious time is. Most of us try to multi task and fit in as much as we can, in the time that we do have. This is an easy to follow guide, which shows you what has basically taken me a lifetime to learn. It will give you the steps to help change your attitude and look at life differently. The strategies will help you surround yourself with people who are loving, positive and supportive. I will show you how to eat normally, lose weight and more importantly keep the weight off. You will also learn how to take control of your money and lead a happy life where you can shop, save and plan for your own future. I am sharing my knowledge from my "own hands" on experience and will demonstrate strategies that have worked in my life. In order to be happier, you must find balance in all areas of your life including relationships, body, and finances.

Relationships

Relationships underpin every area of your life. It is often the reason why we are unhappy and then turn to food or shopping to make ourselves feel better. The most important relationship is the one you have with yourself. This may sound like a cliché but you really do need to start loving yourself first before you can have a happy life. Putting yourself down and believing that you are not good enough leaves an empty hole inside of you. No amount of food or shopping will be able to fill the pain and emptiness you feel. Work on yourself first and be willing to change the way you approach life.

The relationships you have around you also affect your happiness. If you are surrounded by negative, angry and unhappy people, then chances are you will be unhappy. Some of you may find it easy to identify the people who make you feel down. While others may find it hard to identify who is upsetting them. I will show you strategies on how to identify the people who are negative. It does not mean that they are bad people. You just need to work on these relationships so that they are more positive. Your interaction with these people will then be different so that you can turn it into a more positive experience. I know from my own experience, that it is possible to attract more positive people into your life. Life will change and you will see that their positive attitude will also make you feel better.

Body

Today's woman in Western society has more choices now than any woman in known history. She can work, stay home, study, have children or choose not to have children. However this plethora of choices has only added confusion and stress, as women try to figure out what suits them best.

So while it may appear that you have a lot of choices in your lives, you actually have only one choice about what you actually look like. Advertisements in the media, movies and television shows give you only one option of how a woman's body should appear. All women should be skinny and look young, regardless of how old they are. Just turn on your TV or open a magazine and you are bombarded by images of beautiful, young, skinny women.

Young girls are growing up with images of what they "should" look like. This has resulted in an increase in eating disorders amongst our young girls and women. I struggled with an eating disorder when I was younger, so I can imagine that even more girls and women must be struggling with it today. The issues around body image is further exacerbated by shows on plastic surgery. They send the message to females that we have imperfections and that we can fix them by having surgery. It also highlights that we cannot age gracefully and that we need to defy nature and have surgery to make our bodies look better and younger. The hidden message in today's media is telling the females in our society that we are not good enough and that we need to diet, lose weight and have plastic surgery to be attractive and happy.

The pressure to conform to society's view of a beautiful woman has led to girls and women having many issues with their weight and body image. Many people are confused with all the different dietary advice that is available and go on diets, lose the weight but put it all back on over time.

I had issues with my body image from the age of nine; until I discovered how to accept my body and be my ideal weight. If I can do it then you can all do it. I am not asking you to do anything dramatic. You only have to be willing to have an open mind and follow the suggestions in this book. I will teach you how to lose weight and keep it off. Many of you will be amazed at how free and de-stressed you will suddenly feel, now that your life is not ruled by your weight and your body image issues. Once you have let go of your weight issues, you will be able to spend your energy doing more enjoyable things and loving life more freely.

Money

Money is also something that we all need to learn about as it gives us choices in our lives. I am not talking about having more money to buy more "stuff." For instance, would you rather be at work or would you rather be at home with your family or doing something that you love?

The most common stories I have heard again and again, are of women who become divorced or separated and are now finding it financially hard to look after their children and themselves. In fact many women stay in bad marriages due to financial reasons. Most of the time, women have either given up work to stay home or work part time so that they can take care of their children. So when they suddenly find themselves 'alone', they have lost their confidence in working and earning a salary. Looking after children also limits women in the hours they can work and the money they can earn. Suddenly they are living stressful lives as they try to make ends meet.

Many people ignore or think that it is very hard to learn about money or finances. They believe that money is something that professionals or their partners know about, so they leave it others. Unfortunately, only you can take care of yourself financially. If you cannot be bothered looking after your own money, do you honestly believe that someone else is going to do it for you? The answer I am sorry to say is "NO". You need to step up and take responsibility for your own finances.

During my life I have met many women who have had financial issues. Most people have never been taught anything about money. They learn about finances through trial and error, from the first time they receive their pocket money, or when they start working and receive a wage. Then they get a credit card and their journey into debt is sealed. No one has ever explained to them the best way to use a credit card. Yes, there is a good way to use one!

Money can appear to be a "boring subject". However, if you are stressed every day from living in debt, and staring at the countless bills, do you think a lesson in understanding money is boring?

There is also the perception that understanding money is hard. I often hear women say that they are not good with figures. A lot of women found maths difficult at school, so they automatically think that they will be bad at finances or managing money. Surprisingly, it is easy to understand money. Can you add one and one and get two? Can you subtract one from four and get three? Then you are great with money! Money only requires you to add up or subtract. You do not need to do a complicated algebra formula in order to understand money and work out a budget. Anyone can learn about money, you just have to find the motivation and believe that you can understand it.

To show you how I learnt to achieve a much happier lifestyle, I will first tell you a bit about myself and my own struggle with weight and money.

My Story

In this lifetime, I feel that I am here to pass on what I have learnt. Earth is like a classroom and we are here to learn lessons from both our good and bad experiences so that we may grow spiritually.

With this in mind, I will tell you my story from the view point of someone who has experienced a lot and has learnt to feel compassion for those who have been in my life. This has not happened overnight. It has taken a lifetime of soul searching to finally let go of the anger and pain and to replace it with peace and non-judgement.

My issues with weight started at nine years of age when my parents migrated from Malaysia to Australia. In Malaysia, I was a skinny child and never had any issues with my body. However when we moved to Australia, I found that I had put on weight.

Perhaps it was a combination of the different food and the change in climate and culture. The cold weather meant that we stayed indoors more and we ate more "fatty foods" like chocolate biscuits, which were not readily available in Malaysia.

The first time I even realised that I had put on weight was at the age of nine when a family friend named Jenny made the comment that I was "fat" and needed to lose weight. I remember looking at her and saying that she was fat too. Jenny then said that it was alright for her to be overweight, as she was older and married. However since I was young, I needed to be skinny.

This statement hurt and made me feel 'awful' about myself and I did not know what to do with the information. All I knew was that suddenly I was fat and somehow needed to lose weight. There was something wrong with my body and me. This was the start of my weight issues which continued for the next 20 years.

Life was pretty tough in the following years as Jenny repeatedly told me that I was overweight. However, no one ever taught me how to lose the weight, so as I grew older my self-esteem suffered and I felt fat and ugly.

My family also moved around country New South Wales a number of times, before finally settling in

Sydney when I was twelve years old and in the sixth grade. I was one of the tallest people in my grade. No one ever called me fat at school, however I felt big compared to the other children. I recall that towards the end of the sixth grade, it was summer but I refused to take off my bottle green cardigan. I felt that the cardigan hid my fat so I would leave it on even when I was hot. One day my teacher came up to me and forced me to take off my cardigan. I removed it but mentally, I felt 'fat' and uncomfortable.

When I got to high school, there were other kids who were taller and bigger than me, so I did not feel too overweight. No one ever called me fat, so I felt fairly 'normal' in my school uniform. The strange thing was that while at home, I still felt large as Jenny continued to tell me that I needed to lose kilos.

Then one day, when I was fifteen years old, a family friend came to visit and in front of me, he told my parents that I needed to lose weight. This comment from a total stranger crushed me and I became desperate to become skinnier.

Not long after, I watched a TV show about anorexia nervosa and I saw how girls lost weight by making themselves sick or by using diuretics. At the time, I thought I had found the solution to my "weight problem". So after dinner each night, I would make myself sick. The months went by, the kilos slipped off and my family started to pay me compliments. Everyone stopped commenting on my weight, so I was hooked on losing weight in this unhealthy way.

My eating disorder is probably the most difficult part of my life to disclose but I believe it is important to let others know about my own struggles. Hopefully this will inspire them to know that it is an illness you can get over.

My eating disorder lasted for the next ten years of my life and it was like being in hell on earth. Every day for the next ten years, I would wake up in the hope that I would eat well and not binge and purge. However, I failed every single time and this only made me feel worse about myself. I was disgusted and ashamed by my own behaviour and my inability to control it. I kept it a secret from my closest friends.

It amazes me now that despite my illness, I managed to complete high school and graduate from University majoring in Accounting. I say amazes me because when I had bulimia my emotions were erratic, I had dramatic mood swings and my concentration was also affected. The stress from the exams also triggered my eating disorder. I felt as though I was in a deep pit filled with pain the whole time. I focused on food, my weight, exercise, body and eating disorder every minute of every day.

While I was studying, I worked various part time jobs to support myself, so money was very tight. All my money was basically spent, as I lived from pay cheque to pay cheque. I was ecstatic when I graduated and started working in my first full time job. This is when I started to save and budget my money carefully. While studying Accounting at University, I found that it did not show me how to fully understand and make money for myself. This understanding would come from my own research by reading various books and talking to different people.

To my dismay, my eating disorder continued while I was working. I attended the gym every day and tried to eat well, however I continued to suffer from my disorder and I felt like a failure. My family knew I had issues but my friends were oblivious to my condition. Even my best friend from school did not know about my illness, as I was able to hide it from her.

A year and a half after working, I moved to Melbourne and got married. I fell pregnant soon after and realised that I needed to eat well so that my baby would be healthy. My love for my unborn child gave me the strength to take control. So for the first time in ten years, I started to eat properly and my eating disorder disappeared forever. I was 26 years old and I was finally free from a disease that had been controlling me since I was fifteen.

After settling into my family life, I started looking for a way to earn enough income to give me the lifestyle I wanted. In other words, I wanted to spend more time with my family but at the same time maintain or increase the amount of money I was receiving each week. This search led me to property investment, as I was able to understand how it worked. I found the share market was too complicated and unpredictable for my own comfort level. I did my property research and bought my first investment property with my two young children in tow. My partner and I then bought a few investment properties together and all we had to do next was to sit back and wait for the property values to increase. The next step in my long term investment plan was to start doing property developments.

A few years later, my partner and I separated and got divorced. This left me emotionally devastated and I had to reassess everything in my life. I was used to being in a double full time income household. Suddenly I was on a single part time parent income. We sold our joint properties and I started renting for the first time in ten years. The change in life style was both dramatic and traumatic.

I made the decision to work part time, as I wanted to be around to emotionally support my children through the divorce. During the divorce my assets were frozen. My part time wages were going towards rent and childcare and I was surviving on a shoe-string budget. A friend of mine told St Vincent's De Paul about my situation and they appeared one day and handed me food vouchers.

When I was married, I had always donated to charities, but I had never dreamed in a million years that I would ever need charity myself one day. It was a humiliating moment for me but I had to accept it for my children. In another way, it was comforting to see the positive work that charities also carry out, and the kindness provided whilst I was going through a difficult time.

I lost some weight during this period but I was still heavier than my goal weight. No matter how much I exercised, I could not reduce those last few kilos. My whole life felt as though it was in turmoil and I started to question everything. I recall wondering one particular day why it all seemed to be so difficult. Out of coincidence, within the next week, two friends of mine recommended that I read the same book and I took it as a sign and read it. The book was about the law of attraction and it changed my life forever. Funnily enough, both the other women did not get as much out of it as I did.

It showed me how books can be helpful to some and not to others. It is similar to how you can enter a room full of people and only feel comfortable with one person in the whole room. Books are as individual as the people who write them. If you are searching for ways to improve your life, then I encourage you to keep reading books by many authors, to find a book that you identify with.

When I first read about the law of attraction, I was a bit sceptical about the concept. The law of attraction simply states that like attracts like. If you are feeling angry and depressed, then you will attract people and circumstances which will make you feel unhappy. Alternatively if you are happy and positive, then you will attract people and circumstances that make you happy. After reading about the law of attraction and then analysing and applying it to my own life, I found the change in my own life was too noticeable to ignore. Having a positive mindset really did help me make changes in my life that made me feel happier.

Everyone is different and has to make up their mind. I am not here to convert anyone, but simply to share my experiences with others, in the hope that you will get some benefit out of my own life experiences and possibly even feel inspired to change the direction of your life.

I started to think positively about my life, and tried different strategies. By using trial and error, I found out what worked for me. I continued to read other books and over time I found that my life did change for the better.

My children and I are now happier and I live a very content life. I have been able to maintain my weight for years and I continue to eat well and exercise, as it makes me feel good. My financial situation is now back to what it was when I was married. The last few years showed me just how important certain strategies are, in order to have a good relationship with both food and money.

I want to share my strategies with you, as if I can do it, you can too. Everyone deserves to be happy and I hope that this book will change your life for the better.

How to Use this book

You will need to read all the chapters of the book in order. A notebook will also help you work through some of the exercises and help you think about your life. Do not be afraid to jot things down. Throughout the book I will be showing you 'real life' examples, to help you understand the concepts. The examples are taken from women that I have met in my life. They have kindly allowed me to use their stories and I have only changed their names to protect their privacy. These are ordinary women who have overcome some difficult issues and would like to share their life lessons with you.

Chapter One focuses on you and makes recommendations of what you can do to make yourself happy. You will not be able to make changes to the other areas of your life if you are tired and stressed. Look after yourself first and then you will have the energy to make changes in the other areas of your life.

Chapter Two looks at all the relationships in your life and allows you to decide how you want to handle them, so that they are more positive. You will need a notebook or piece of paper to write down your answers.

Chapter Three is written in a step by step sequence. In order to lose weight and keep it off, you need to follow each step as set out in the book.

Chapter Four is also written in a step by step sequence. You will need a notebook and calculator so that you can work out your own budget. Stop getting stressed and being worried. Remember you are not being asked to do algebra or some other complicated maths. You only have to add up, take away, multiply and divide. All of these can be done using a calculator. It is easy and it will help you have more money in your life.

Chapter Five summaries what has been discussed in the previous chapters. So you can use it to refresh your memory after you have read the whole book. Life now can be better than your past. What happened to you before can be left behind. You can make the changes you need so that you can be happy now for both you and your family. Good luck and remember every woman deserves to feel good!

Chapter 1

Looking after yourself

Positive intentions are the stepping stones to a happier life

In order for you to be happier you need to be willing to change the way you approach life. You need to first start by looking after yourself. Stress from your daily life will affect your mental and physical health. Continually doing things for other people and ignoring your own needs is only going to make you unhappy and depressed in the long term. If you do not look after yourself you will not be able to live your life to the fullest or have the energy to support your family.

Many women feel emptiness inside and they try to fill the hole with romantic relationships, food or shopping. They then find that they have problems in all three areas. You may not even realise that you feel this way. Here are simple ways to help you improve the relationship you have with yourself and change your attitude towards life.

Step 1—Realising that everyone has problems and you have the power to decide how you are going to react to the problem.

Everyone has problems in their life, just look at your circle of friends. Do any of them have any problems? You will find that they will all say yes. So you are not the only person in the world with issues. Every person on the planet has problems.

I used to drop off my youngest son to childcare on the way to work. Every morning I would see another mum drop her two young kids off around the same time. We would both smile and say hello to one another. She always wore a smart looking business suit, she had long blonde hair, a great figure and as you can imagine was very attractive. I was going through my own divorce at that stage and would look at this woman with tinges of envy. She looked as though she had everything in her life sorted. I imagined that her husband was a professional Executive, as well and that the two of them led comfortable lives.

Then one day we started to have a brief chat and I found out that her name was Emma and that I was wrong about her perfect life. Sadly, her husband had cheated on her with another woman while she was pregnant with their second child. He left and has refused to see their children. Furthermore, Emma was also having trouble trying to get him to pay child support. She was going through a tough time and not leading the perfect life I had imagined. I realised that day that everyone has problems, even the ones who look as though they have a perfect life.

Instead of dwelling on your problems, you have to change *your* attitude towards them. A lot of the times things happen to us which are beyond our control. Instead of feeling upset and powerless, you have to realise that you can control your reaction to the problem. You get to decide how you are going to react to the situation.

In Emma's case she did not quit her job and stay home complaining about the problems in her life. She continued to work and carried on living. You could tell from the way she spoke, that she had a positive attitude and was making the most of her situation.

Step 2—Be grateful for what you have

Given that we all have problems, it is important to change the way we think and focus on the positive areas of our lives. We have to change our mindset altogether. One way to help you feel better about your life, is to be grateful every day for the little things in it. Yes there are good things in your life. We are lucky to be living in a country free from war; we have electricity, and clean water to drink. Not everyone in this world is so lucky. There are millions of people around the world who are starving, live in war zones, do not have electricity or clean water. You need to realise how blessed you are and be grateful for the little things in your life that you do have. Focusing on the good things in your life will draw more positive experiences to you.

Step 3—You cannot change your past, so focus on your future

The next concept that you have to understand is that you cannot change what has happened in your past. You have to make the decision today to stop dwelling on the bad things that have happened to you. Focus on what is happening now and then think about your future. Tomorrow is a blank canvas and you can create whatever you want. Always remember that you may have had a tough past, but you get to decide what happens to your future. You are the only one who can choose to have a better future.

Some people blame their parents for their problems now. You may have had a tough or even abusive childhood however your parents did the best they could. They may have also had a difficult childhood so they did not have the skills to nurture you in a positive way. Your parents are only human and you have to try and let go of any anger or resentment you have towards them.

The life you now lead is your responsibility. You cannot use the excuse of what happened to you ten years ago for what is happening in your life now. Draw a line in the sand and see a counsellor if necessary to help you move on with your life. When you keep thinking about all the negative things that happened to you, there is no opportunity to move on and you will continue to harbour resentments and attract negativity into your life. You deserve to be happy now, so let go of your past.

Annabel divorced Jason after ten years of marriage. They had married and after two years they began their family. Over the next eight years they had three beautiful children Leanne, Oscar and Kyra. They decided together that Annabel would stay home as the primary care giver, while the children grew up. Annabel gave up her career as a lawyer to focus on her family. During their ten year marriage, Annabel and Jason had their ups and downs. Jason was also a lawyer and worked long hours, travelling interstate and overseas frequently. After ten years of marriage they began to drift apart, and this led to the divorce.

Their separation was amicable and their assets were divided satisfactorily between the two of them.

Five years after their divorce, however, Annabel was still not satisfied as she remained at home looking after her children. Jason continued in his career and was now moving in with his new partner. He appeared to be doing much better financially than Annabel. During the five years after her divorce, Annabel had focused on the decision to put her career on hold, to look after her family. She kept focusing on the past and on all the things she had missed out on. Her friends and family were constantly listening to her complain about the mistakes she had made in her past. Then one day her daughter Leanne, who was now a teenager decided to set her mother straight. "You know mum, we all appreciated you being around for us when we were younger. We have all grown up now so why don't you get back to work and focus on your career?". That simple comment from her daughter made Annabel look at her life again and she realised that she could start a new career. She decided to start a business and she opened a café. Two years later Annabel is happier and her business is booming. She stopped focusing on her past and took action to have a better future. The morale of the story is that we all need to let go of our past in order to move forward.

Step 4—Whatever you focus on, will come true

Whatever we focus on will come true, whether we want it or do not want it. It is amazing how our beliefs actually create the circumstances in our life. Kate grew up in a household where there was domestic violence. Her parents fought constantly and her father was violent and occasionally hit her mother and siblings. Kate was very unhappy as a child and hated the fact that her family seemed to be so dysfunctional. When she grew into a teenager she decided that she was not going to marry an abusive man who would hurt her or her children. Kate grew up, finished school and then met James. He was so romantic and within the first few weeks of meeting each other, he told Kate how much he loved her. They spent all their time together and Kate fell hopelessly in love with James. She kept watching James' behaviour to see if he was violent or abusive, but James was always loving. When they had fights, they would say awful things to each other and then make up later. James was so sensitive that he would even cry when they fought. Kate thought that James was romantic, as he kept buying her gifts and flowers. He had a younger brother whom he looked after and was very close to. James' behaviour caused Kate to believe that she had met a loving and gentle man. A year after they met, Kate and James walked down the aisle and got married. Within a year of the wedding, Kate fell pregnant. She was overjoyed by the news as she always wanted to be a mum. However, James did not seem happy and the man that Kate had married started to change. James would get angry and he started to get violent and verbally abusive. He started to throw things when they argued and eventually Kate started to fear him. She realised that she had married a man that was exactly like her father. They were controlling, violent and abusive men. Kate eventually left James as she found that he was growing more angry and abusive.

Looking back at her life, Kate realised that she had attracted James into her life because she had been focusing on an abusive man. It did not matter that she was asking for the opposite. The fact that she was thinking about an abusive man, drew James into her life.

After her divorce, Kate focused on making herself happier and changing her mindset. She eventually met a kind and loving man named Paul. They dated for a few years before eventually getting married. Five years later, Paul was still the same kind and loving man that she had first met. Kate had focused on what she had wanted this time and her dreams were answered.

Step 5—Does judging others make anyone happy?

It is amazing how I hear people complain about someone else's behaviour, yet they or their own immediate family members, have behaved in exactly the same behaviour that they are complaining about. Before you start to judge others, look in the mirror and reflect on yourself. Why are the other person's actions affecting you? Can you recognise some of their behaviour in yourself? What can you change about yourself so that you are the person you want to be around? Would you want other people to gossip about you in the same way that you are talking about them?

Janet was complaining to her friend Simone that people at her work gossiped a lot. That she was sick of their behaviour and that they should be focusing on their work and not everyone else's private lives.

The very next day Janet saw two people kissing in the staff car park and realised that it was Tom and Sally from her work. Tom was married and Janet realised that he was having an affair with Sally. When Janet got into the office she started to tell one of her work mates about Tom and Sally kissing in the car park. Half way through her conversation, she realised that she was doing exactly what she had been complaining about. She was gossiping about her work mates.

We all judge other people but you can start to change that attitude once you can recognise it in yourself. Before you start to point the finger at other people's behaviour, look at you own actions. Next time just observe what is around you without judgement of others or yourself.

Step 6—Learning from your bad experiences

During your life, like most people, you would have had both positive and negative experiences. All experiences have the potential to help you grow and be a stronger person. When you survive a particularly troubled time, it shows you just how strong you really are. In future, when something upsetting happens in your life, give yourself time to deal with the issue and then get over the event. You have to realise that you are a resilient person for surviving the experience. Then try and see what lesson you can learn from the experience and move on.

Leslie was looking for a financial advisor and she saw an advertisement for an investment company in the local newspaper. So she made an appointment and met Robert who was one of the advisors in the company. When Leslie first met Robert she had an uneasy feeling about him. Her inner voice told her not to trust him. However Robert was very charming and by the end of the meeting, Leslie had signed a contract to invest some of her money with Robert's company. When Leslie left the office she started to have second thoughts and regretted signing the contract. Something did not feel right about Robert. However after speaking to her friends, she convinced herself that it was just nerves and ignored her feelings.

Six months later Leslie lost all the money that she had invested with Robert. The company contacted her, to alert her that Robert had stolen the money from a number of his clients and had left the country. Leslie was devastated and it took her a few months to get over her anger at Robert and losing her money. Over time Leslie realised that she should have trusted her own gut instinct about Robert, instead of allowing herself to be influenced by Robert's smile and nice manners.

After this awful experience, Leslie started to educate herself by reading books and talking to different people about investing and money. She realised that understanding finances was not as difficult as she had always imagined.

Two years later, a friend of Leslie's told her about a financial planner named Rebecca who was supposed to be very good. Leslie met Rebecca and this time, she paid attention to how she felt about Rebecca when she first met her. After listening to Rebecca's sale pitch, Leslie was able to see that Rebecca's figures and logic did not make sense. The alarm bells went off and this time Leslie listened to her inner voice. She left the office and told Rebecca that she was not interested. Leslie eventually started managing her own investments and made more money than she had lost several years ago. A year later Leslie found out that Rebecca had made some bad decisions and lost some of her client's money, including her friends.

Leslie realised that she might have had one bad experience but it had taught her to trust her own gut instinct about people. It had also motivated her to improve her knowledge about investing and money, so that she can look after her own future.

Step 7—Help comes from many places, so accept it when it is offered

No one is ever really alone. Sometimes your immediate family may not be supportive of you but you have friends or even strangers who are there to give you the support you need. Think back now to a situation when you were going through a really bad time. Who was around you? Sometimes there are people who are waiting to help you. However you may have chosen to reject their advice or support. So the next time you are going through a particularly bad time, accept help when it is offered. You do not have to go through life alone. Open your eyes and look around you. What I am saying is that you are never truly alone or left to deal with issues by yourself. Help and support is there even though it might not come in the form you expect.

Aliyah and her children moved to Perth for her work. She had left all her family behind in her home town of Melbourne. Aliyah did not know anyone in Perth and was very nervous about how she was going to survive by herself. After a few months Aliyah met Sally when she took her kids to the school fete. Sally was also divorced and she and Aliyah got along as soon as they met each other.

One day Aliyah's son Nathan fell down and broke his ankle. He normally walked to and from school himself as Aliyah worked full time. At first Aliyah started crying and stressing out about how she was going to work, if she had to take Nathan to school and pick him up. However, after a sleepless night, Aliyah decided to ask Sally for help. As soon as Aliyah explained that Nathan had hurt his ankle, Sally immediately volunteered to take Nathan to school. Aliyah was relieved as she could now go to work and know that Nathan would be looked after by Sally.

We are never really alone and the right people always come into our lives to help us. You just have to be open to it and be thankful for their support.

Step 8—Forgive and forget

In your life you may have encountered people who have hurt you in one way or another. However, you have to learn not to take on their issues. You cannot change the person who has hurt you or their behaviour towards you. The only thing you can change is your attitude towards them. So it is important to focus on that and forgive and forget. Remembering the bad things that someone has done to you, will only make you unhappy. Allow yourself a time period in which to heal and then change your focus to making yourself happier. You need to take back your power and not let the people who have hurt you in the past, to take away your future happiness.

In the story in step 6 Leslie lost money by ignoring her own gut instinct and investing her money with Robert. At the beginning Leslie was very angry and kept talking about Robert to her friends. She could not believe how Robert could lie and steal her money. One day Leslie was at the beach and decided that it was time to let go of her anger towards Robert. She mentally threw her anger into the water and promised herself that she would stop talking about Robert from that day on. Leslie was surprised at how lighter she felt once she had let go of her anger. Robert may have stolen her money and in a sense her trust towards other people. However, Leslie did not allow him to affect her future by carrying around her anger.

Step 9—Karma

My interpretation of the word 'karma' is that what energy you put out comes back to you. Another saying is 'what goes around comes around'. When you behave in a positive way, you attract positive energy. Alternatively, when you behave negatively, you attract negative energy. I have seen this happen in my life as well as the lives of other people. If you look around, you will also see evidence of this with people you know.

Years ago I had a Manager who was very ambitious and would do anything to get to the top of the organisation. He was very manipulative, lied and twisted facts to "manage" people. It appeared as though the organisation looked at him as a future leader. His unethical behaviour however, eventually caught up with him. Years later, I found out that he was demoted due to a mild heart attack and was divorced. Basically his whole life fell apart. I realised that due to his actions his whole life turned upside down. He reaffirmed for me that people do get back what they put out. It may not happen straight away but it will happen eventually. Unfortunately he never made the connection with his behaviour to what happened in his life.

So now when people do not live up to your expectations, just walk away. Life is too short to hold grudges against anyone. The only person you hurt is yourself. When things happen, I now look at what I learnt from that experience, and then move on. Life is a journey and we are here to develop ourselves. Others have to take responsibility for their own actions. Let's face it, some people go through a whole life time and never realise how their actions will eventually affect others or themselves.

The bible tells us to love our neighbours like thyself because it understands that whatever energy you put out, comes back to you. So if you have strong negative feelings against someone like anger, then you will have negative energy returning to you. Loving your enemy may be hard and probably unrealistic for most of us. So I have found that blessing people actually removes the negativity. Blessing is the opposite of cursing. You are basically wishing someone well, and that positive energy will be returned to you. I have been amazed at how circumstances change as soon as you bless someone. It is amazing how people suddenly change the way they treat you. You can then let go of any negative emotions and enjoy your life.

Jessie was having trouble with her manager at work. No matter what she did, her manager was always criticising her work. Jessie dreaded going to work and having to deal with him. It made her moody and grumpy and as a result she became known at work as the one with the bad attitude. Then one day she read about blessing people and having nothing to lose, Jessie started to bless her manager. Whenever she saw, thought about or interacted with her boss, she would mentally say "I bless you." At first nothing happened but after a few days Jessie noticed that he was not criticising her as much. Over the next few months, Jessie was able to shift her attitude to work, so that she was no longer feeling negative about it. To her surprise, a new Manager from a different section noticed Jessie's positive attitude and experience, and offered her a promotion to his area. Jessie could not believe her luck and accepted the new position. By changing her attitude, Jessie was now seen as a positive worker and was able to gain a better position.

Step 10—Focus on being happy <u>now</u>

When you go through challenging experiences in your life, it is not surprising that you will get affected both emotionally and physically. You have to heal and the only person who can help you heal, is yourself. The best way to heal yourself is to allow yourself a period of time where you feel the pain and hurt. Then after a period, make the decision that you have to go on with your life and start doing things that bring you joy.

Dwelling on your bad experiences for long periods of time will eventually have a negative effect on all areas of your life. You may get sick or your relationships start to have problems. Depression and a range of other mental illnesses may also develop.

I have learnt that you do not have to be the victim. Everything that happened to you in the past, can be mentally left behind. Your life now and your future, is in your control and what you want to make of it.

When you are happy, it is amazing just how good you start to feel and this helps you heal faster. There are times when things are not perfect but you can make the effort to steer yourself back to focusing on the positive. Remember there are people in this world who live in countries with war and famine. You are in a fortunate position if you have clean water to drink, a safe place to sleep and food in the cupboard.

Rani had grown up in a violent household and she did not have a good relationship with her parents. When Rani left home, she kept thinking about her past and the pain she had gone through. She was full of anger and could not move past her abusive childhood. The years went by and Rani found herself in one bad relationship after another, with negative, abusive and angry men. Eventually she went and had counselling and started to let go of her past. She realised that even though she was physically a thirty two year old woman, her thoughts were still that of the little girl who was angry at her parents. Rani blessed her parents whenever she found herself thinking about them. She also read books and attended seminars and over time, her past faded into the background. Instead of waiting for Mr Right to enter her life before she could be happy, Rani made the decision that she would start to be happy from now. She focused on enjoying her photography and travelling. Her new passion for life meant that she stopped wanting to hang around angry and depressed people, who made her feel uncomfortable. Now she preferred people who had a passion for living and did not sit around complaining. Rani eventually met a loving and caring man, who shared her interest in photography.

Rani learnt that she had everything to gain, by forgetting about her past and just enjoying life now.

Step 11—Activities to remove stress and make you feel good

Imagine your energy is in a bucket of water. Every time you look after your family, or go to work, you are using up the water in the bucket. If you do not take the time to stop and fill up your bucket, then you will be empty. Once you are empty, you cannot give any more to anyone else. You become tired, exhausted and will not have any energy to look after your family or work. So you need to look after yourself.

Here are a number of ways to recharge your spirit:

1) **Reading personal development books or watching dvds**—The library and book stores have a great selection under their self-development sections. There are many authors so try and find one that you can relate to.
2) **Counselling**—It is so important that you find the right counsellor. Your needs will also change over time. So a counsellor that helped you for a certain period of time may not be suitable at a later stage. Please remember

that just because a person calls themselves a counsellor or psychologist does not mean that they are always right. **Always go with your gut instinct**!! If your stomach churns because of something they have asked you to do, then this is a warning for you to take a step back, evaluate the situation a bit further before making a final decision. The counsellor is only there to help you cope with the stresses in your life. They are not there to make decisions about legal and financial matters.

3) **Staying positive**—Read books, and watch movies that make you laugh. The happier you are, the more happiness will come to you.

4) **What are you waiting for? Be happy now**—You do not have to wait for the troubles in your life to go away before you believe you can be happy. In fact the reverse is true. If you are happy now, you will find that your troubles will go away. Just try it yourself by focusing on the things and people that make you happy now. Start being happy now and watch your troubles disappear.

5) **Surround yourself with friends and family who support you**—There is a saying which goes something like this "Birds of a feather flock together." This basically means that you attract people who are like you. So look around at your friends, as that is the type of person you are. What type of people are they?

Are they positive? Are they negative? Do they make you feel good? Do they make you feel bad? If they make you feel bad, you will have to distance yourself from these people, as you will find that they are unhappy themselves and that the only way they feel better about themselves is to criticize you. Any person who criticizes you and "makes you **feel bad**" is not a true friend. Some of these people may even be immediate family members. When you start to say no to the negative friends and family, you will find that you will start to attract new and positive people, who will make you happy. This will be discussed further in the relationships chapter.

6) **Do things that make you feel bliss**—To help you bring more happiness into your life here are some suggestions on how to make your life joyful. Everyone is different and so will need to find an activity that interests them.

- Meditation. Have you ever sat quietly and let your mind relax? After a stressful day it is great to sit down quietly, close your eyes and let your mind be still. If you are new to meditating, there are plenty of meditation cds which offer guided meditations. It can be guided meditations where a voice leads you through it. They can include music, voices or bells so that your mind is relaxed. When you are going through an especially difficult time such as a divorce, meditating is a great way to help you calm down. It helps you to take your mind off your worries and be at peace during your meditation. If you happen to fall asleep during your meditation, do not feel as though you have failed. Your body obviously needed the rest. Just keep trying and you will eventually come to look forward to them. You do not have to meditate for long periods of time. It is better to have a good ten minute meditation than to sit for an hour having a frustrated one. There are plenty of classes, dvds and cds to show you how to meditate.

- Yoga is another great way to relax your mind and increase the flexibility of your body. Like meditation there are classes, dvds and cds to show you how to do it. So if you work or have children and you come home late, you can actually practice yoga late at night in front of your tv. It is a great way to make you feel more positive and happier.

- Walking is a great way to get fit without putting too much stress on your body. You can go as fast or as slow as you want. However it is probably better to walk faster than your normal relaxed pace. It is free and all you need is a pair of comfortable shoes. Walking helps to clear your mind and also lift your energy and mood to a more positive level. I found that when you feel down, a quick 30 minute walk lifts your mood up straight away.

- I have named three forms of exercises but the list is endless. Any form of exercise will lift your energy and spirit. The main thing is that you enjoy doing it so that it does not turn into a chore.

- Art is great way to help lift your spirit and look at the beauty there is in the world. You do not have to be able to draw or paint to explore art. You can use a camera to capture the beauty that you see around you. When you start to focus on the beautiful things, a new world suddenly opens up. You will notice things that you have never noticed before. For instance I take the freeway to work and was normally so focused on getting through the traffic that I had never looked around me. Then I started to draw and one day I noticed the beautiful green farms that surrounded the freeway. The cattle were dotted across the fields and the whole scene looked as though it belonged in a painting. Yet I had travelled on the freeway a hundred times previously and had never noticed such beauty around me. Noticing the simple and beautiful things around you, will help to make you feel better and more positive about the world.

- Self-esteem is the way we view and think about ourselves. It is basically how much you feel you are worth as a person. A lot of us have had experiences which makes us feel that we are not good enough. Our inner voice is constantly telling us negative things about ourselves. Just sit there for a moment and write a description of yourself. Are the words positive or negative? Examples of low self-esteem are "I am fat and ugly", "I am stupid", "I hate my teeth". If you are always saying or thinking negative thoughts about yourself then you have low self-esteem. The good news is that you can improve it, so that you will feel good about yourself.

Jasmine grew up in a household where she was constantly criticised and made to feel that she had a lot problems. That she was a girl who was overweight and unattractive. So Jasmine grew up with very low self-esteem and feeling as though she was never good enough. Unfortunately this low self-esteem led Jasmine into unhealthy relationships. Her inner voice kept reinforcing to Jasmine that no one else would love her, so she had to stay with her current partner. After several unsuccessful relationships Jasmine decided to see a counsellor and work on her self-esteem. During that year she remained single and did activities that made her feel good about herself. She learned to accept herself and love her beautiful red hair and porcelain skin. A year later Jasmine is a new woman. She is now confident and feels good about herself and she has found that she is attracting very different people into her life. Her circle of friends has widened and she is much happier.

- Doing a short course that interests you is a great way to help you clear your mind and make you feel better. When you focus on something that you have to learn, you will find that it will make you feel better and expand your mind.

    Leslie, a friend of mine, had overcome some major issues in her life. Then one day she woke up feeling depressed and could not understand why she was feeling so low. On the face of it, everything in her life was going well with her family and work. Leslie then took a course in photography and suddenly she felt more positive. She found something that she enjoyed and it had helped her recharge her 'battery'. Learning something that you enjoy will help you exercise your mind and feel good.

- All of us are different so you need to find an activity that you can do, to help you lift your mood. This list is not exhaustive and since everyone is different, you can experiment until you find something that makes you happy. It is possible to feel happier in your life and you can do it.

    A friend of mine named Mary once said to me that she felt guilty for being happy in her relationship, as one of her good friends, Erin, was having a lot of problems. We are responsible for our own lives. Mary can listen to Erin's problems but she does not need to feel guilty about being happy in her own life. We are all responsible for our own happiness.

Step 12—Surround yourself with happy people

There are certain "friends" who can make you feel bad and a bit flat. They make comments that make you feel bad about yourself. There are also other friends who are so negative that they always seem depressed. Nothing you do can help them feel better. They also seem to absorb your energy so that you are left feeling tired and drained after spending time with them.

These type of people make you feel bad and you will never be happy if you have negative people around you. Surround yourself with happy (most of the time) people, and you will find that they will help you maintain your happiness.

Step 13—Beauty comes from within

When you start being happy and positive you will notice that people will start to think that you look different, younger and more attractive. Beauty radiates from within and if you are happy on the inside then it will show on the outside. Think about some of the people that you have met. When you think of the people who are always just mean spirited, angry and generally negative, what do they look like? Do you like being around them? Now think of the people who are happy, always laughing and are generally positive. Are they attractive? Do you like them? Your face reflects your thoughts and feelings. If you are unhappy on the inside, then your face will show it.

Step 14—Help other people

It is important that we help others if we can. When we help other people, the energy you put out comes back to help you as well. The more people you help, the more positive energy comes back to you.

When I help someone, I feel good that it has made a difference in their life. It might only be a small gesture but I still feel happy that I was able to assist that person. The person I helped also feels good. So the happy feeling you created comes back to you twice. The more people you help, the more positive energy comes back to you.

Even if you cannot understand what I am saying, go out and do a good deed for someone else. The very act of helping other people will make you feel good. It does not need to be anything big, the smallest act can make a difference in a person's life.

Years ago I had to do a presentation at work. I checked my notebook several times and made sure that it worked. Unfortunately on the day of the presentation, something went wrong with the sound on my notebook. I got so stressed until another colleague named Angela, had a look at it and fixed the problem. I was able to do my presentation and it went well. I was so happy and grateful for Angela's help. This happened over ten years ago but I still remember the help that Angela gave me that day.

So whenever you can, try and help the people around you. It will help you feel good and make you a happier person.

Step 15—Respect your body

This part relates to women who feel bad about themselves and try to feel better by having regular casual sex or one night stands. If you are happy with yourself, then you do not have to listen to what I am saying. I am not judging you or trying to 'preach'. What I am saying is that if you are feeling bad about yourself, then casual sex is not going to make you feel better about yourself. Yes we are living in modern times where there is equality between the sexes. If you are looking for a relationship then having sex with a man too early in the relationship may cause you to lose him. Take your time to know him as a person and you can then decide if you want him in your life. Your body is special and you need to be choosy about who you allow near it. Just think about your own house or apartment. Would you allow a total stranger to make themselves at home by using your lounge room, bathroom and kitchen? Your body is more valuable than any place you live in.

Think about the emotions you feel after you have casual sex. Do you feel good or bad? Do you feel like running away from the person? Does he want to run away from you? How does that make you feel? What do you do afterwards? Do you eat or shop? Be honest with yourself and think about the answers to the questions above and make up your own mind. No one is judging you. This is about you looking at your behaviour and making the decisions that make you feel truly good about yourself.

Looking after yourself

You are the only person who can look after yourself. In order for you to look after everyone, you need to look after your needs first. So look at your life and start doing a bit of 'house' cleaning. The strategies

I have given you will help to make positive changes in your life. People who are truly joyful, positive and laugh constantly will lead much healthier and fuller lives. You just have to do a bit of 'house' cleaning in your life and look at life differently.

It has taken me a long time to realise that only I can make myself happy. More importantly, how to make myself happy and I hope this helps you to realise that you have the power to do it. Life is meant to be joyous; you just have to believe that you can be happy now.

Chapter 2

Relationships

When you are having problems with food and money, you will discover that the main reason for these problems is that there is something in your life that is making you feel bad. It took me years of soul searching and trying different strategies to make that connection. To show you how to deal with these issues, we need to go back to the basics and that is to look at what is making you feel **bad or unhappy**. You cannot lose weight and keep it off, or manage your finances properly, until you are able to deal with some of the 'triggers' that make you unhappy and depressed. Some of you may not even realise what your trigger is and this is especially true if you have spent most of your life being unhappy and you believe that it is 'normal' and that there is nothing wrong.

When I was in the midst of my eating disorder in my late teens and early twenties, I was depressed. However, I did not know I was depressed at the time, as I had been feeling that way for most of my life. I was also struggling with trying to control my eating disorder and it is only now, when I look back at my life during that period, that I realise I was a very angry and depressed person. The trigger for my unhappiness, I now realise, was my attitude and the negative relationships in my life. These relationships made me feel bad and they contributed to my issues with weight. I did not recover from my eating disorder until I dealt with the relationships that made me feel bad.

Happiness

So what is happiness and how do you know if you are unhappy? One way to find out what happiness 'feels' like, is to think of all the things that make you feel good. For instance, it might have been your 16th birthday party or the time your football team won a game. The way you felt about those events is the feeling of happiness and feeling good. If you are not sure, then grab a journal or diary and write down how you are feeling every day.

Diary or journal

Keeping a diary of what you do and how different things make you feel, is a great way for you to see what is actually happening in your life. Most of us are so busy rushing through our days that we never sit back and reflect on how it was. A diary is a great tool in monitoring how you feel and it shows you how your life is progressing. Sometimes when you see things in writing it is a bit of a wakeup call, especially if you notice that most of the events in your day made you angry or stressed.

A diary is also a great way to find out how your relationships with different people make you feel. In brackets write down how you felt while you were with the person and after you left the person. You can also write down why you felt a certain way after being with that person.

An example of a diary entry is:

Caught up with Jan and Samantha and we went to the beach. (I felt bad as Jan kept ignoring me and only speaking to Samantha)

Remember this is only an example and you can write down as much or as little as you want. The main goal is to work out how different people in your life make you feel, even if you have only met them for the first time.

What makes you happy?

Your unhappiness could be caused by a number of different factors and each person is different. To help you find out what is making you unhappy, I will show you various ways of identifying what is making you feel bad.

Are relationships making you unhappy?

The first possible cause of your unhappiness could be your relationships with your partner, family, friends, work colleagues or anyone else in your life.

You may be one of the few who can easily identify what is making you feel empty and unhappy inside. Unfortunately most of us only notice the image in the mirror, the tightness of our clothes or the amount on our credit card statement. We do not realise that we are unhappy and that there is something missing in our lives. You may believe that you have a bad day occasionally. Unfortunately the issue may be much deeper and harder to solve. So take a piece of paper and write your name in the middle of the page. Put the names of all the people you have contact with in your life. This will make sure you have thought about every person or relationship you have. Always include your immediate family such as your parents and siblings even if you have minimal contact with them.

Here is an example of what to do and I am using Jenny as an example.

Jenny is a happily married mum with two children. She acknowledges that when she has a fight with her husband Gary, she consoles herself with some chocolate. Yes she is overweight and if Jenny was happy with her weight then that is fine, however she is miserable that she is the heaviest she has ever been. Her credit card bill is also large, being one of the reasons why she and her husband Gary have been fighting so much lately. She cannot seem to control her weight or her spending. To help Jenny feel better about her weight and finances we have to start by looking at the relationships in Jenny's life.

Jenny is married to Gary, so she writes Gary's name on the piece of paper with an arrow pointing back to her. Next are Jenny's two children Jasmine and Caleb, so she draws an arrow from her kids and back to herself. Then there are Jenny's work colleagues, some of whom she has a lot to do with, while she has minimal contact with others. So Jenny puts down the names of the people that she has to interact with. Then there is Jenny's parents, brother, sister and friends.

Sample Diagram

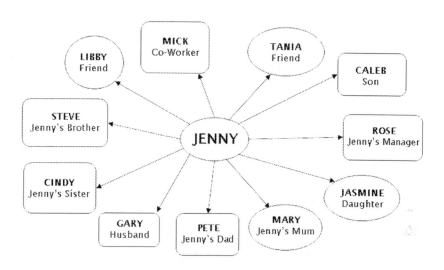

Once Jenny has written down the names of all the people she knows, she needs to write down how each person makes her feel. Do they make her feel good, bad or indifferent? You only need to write down one word and if you are unsure then write down unsure. This is where your diary will be useful in finding out how people make you feel.

To Jenny's surprise she finds that her mother make her feel bad, not Gary, as she had first suspected. When Jenny looks at her diary she realises that her mother never seems to be happy with whatever she does. Jenny sees her parents, Mary and Pete, nearly every weekend as they live only two streets away. The more Jenny thinks about it, the more she realises that she and Gary seem to fight only on the weekends, after she comes home from her parents.

After this realisation, Jenny decides that she is going to start to monitor how she feels whenever she visits her parents. The following weekend, Jenny's mother Mary lets her in and they go into the kitchen to have a coffee. After half an hour, Jenny realises that Mary, keeps making little comments which puts her down. The first comment was that Jenny's new hair style did not suit her. Yet Jenny had left the hair dresser that day feeling like a million dollars. She had been feeling really attractive and happy, until Mary had made the comment. Mary then told Jenny that she was not feeding her children healthy food and that they were too skinny. This made Jenny feel like an awful mother. Next came the complaint about her own husband Pete and this lasted for the rest of her visit. Jenny loved her father and felt upset at having to listen to her mother talk about him. However Jenny knew that she could not say anything to her mother about it, as she would be accused of taking her father's side. When Jenny left her mum's that day she was feeling tired and drained of her energy. She felt like buying some chocolate on her way home, so she stopped at the shopping centre. On her way to the supermarket, she spotted a shop which had a sale and walked into it. By the time Jenny went home, she had purchased chocolates, shoes and a dress she did not really need. When she entered the house, Gary saw the shopping bags and they then started to argue.

Jenny grew up with her mother, so she had not realised that she made her feel bad until now. A lot of us have people in our lives that have been around us for a long time. So you accept them and you do not even realise that they make you feel bad about yourself. You may interact with them occasionally or every day, but unless you make a conscious effort to observe how they make you feel, you never fully realise the impact that they have on you.

In Jenny's case, she has decided to talk to Mary and tell her how she makes her feel. However, you may find that conversation too difficult, so you might decide to reduce the time you spend with that person. Or you could just ignore the negative comments from that person, although this can be hard if the comments really hurt. It all depends on you and your relationship with that person. The bottom line is that if you find that the person makes you feel bad about yourself, then you have to decide how you are going to deal with that person.

The following are some examples of possible negative relationships in your life which are making you feel bad. Remember some of them are hard to spot as they have been in your lives for a long time. The only way you are going to be able to identify them is to observe and think about how people in your life make YOU feel.

The Complainer

The complainer is a person who contacts you and talks about their problems. They may have problems in their romantic relationships or it may be another of their friends. However, the complainer will ring and talk on and on about how bad this person behaved towards them. They are not there to listen to any advice that you may have to offer. Their sole purpose is to complain about people to you. If you are happy to listen to them, then that is fine. However, if you find that they are draining your energy and you feel tired after interacting with them, then you need to start to see less of them. It may also be an idea to meet with them in public places so that they are unable to drain you too much. Another suggestion may be to make excuses that you have another appointment that you have to go to, so that you have limited time with them. Some complainers are genuinely seeking your help as they are trying to leave a bad relationship. If you can see that they are taking some of your advice and you do not feel drained by them, then you may feel comfortable in having them in your life.

Sally rang Cassie every other day to complain about her boyfriend Richard. Whenever Richard did something to upset Sally she was texting or ringing Cassie. Cassie could see that Richard was mistreating Sally. So Cassie eventually told Sally that she needed to leave Richard. Sally agreed at the time but a few days later Sally was back with Richard as he had apologised. Then a week later there was another problem and Sally was back on the phone crying about the latest bad thing that Richard had done. Some people only want to complain and they have no intentions of improving their circumstances. They can drain you of your energy and leave you feeling very tired. It is up to you if you want these types of people in your life. If you value your relationship with that friend then tell them that you are happy to see them, but you refuse to discuss their problem. Then leave it up to your friend as to whether she still wants to see you.

The Energy Sappers

The energy sappers are different from the complainers in that they do not necessarily complain about anything but you feel tired and drained after spending time with them. They are usually depressed but always seem to feel better after spending time with you. The trouble is that while they may feel good, you are left tired and drained. Once again it is up to you as to how you deal with this type of person. You may have to reduce the time you spend with them.

While I was going through my divorce I became friends with a lady named Donna. She was an attractive woman and she seemed really nice and friendly. However, Donna was depressed about her ex-boyfriend and the fact that she was single. She was literally broke and at the age of fifty she only owned her car. I would go out for dinner or coffee with Donna, and try to make her feel better. Then after a while I noticed that after I left Donna, I would feel very tired and drained. It took me a few months to realise that Donna was draining me of my energy. She would feel good after we met, while I felt exhausted. Over time this friendship ended and I now make sure that I have little contact with people who drain me and make me feel bad.

The jealous or envious one

These are people who make comments that make you realise that they are jealous or envious of you. They do not always make you feel unhappy but you are aware that they are not encouraging you to be successful.

Kira was talking to her best friend Lisa about her new boyfriend Josh. Then suddenly Lisa made the comment "Why is it that you seem to meet the really great guys?" The comment by Lisa shows that she does not think that she is able to meet a "great guy". There are in fact plenty of great guys out there and you will meet them if you believe it. However the comment also shows that Lisa is envious of Kira. The situation gets worse when Lisa tries to seduce Kira's boyfriend. You need to be able to trust the people in your life. Look around at your circle of friends and see if you can trust them. If there is any doubt, then you have to decide if you want people like that in your life. Just be aware though, that if you cannot trust the person, then chances are they are making you feel bad.

The abusive/controlling one

The abusive one usually relates to a romantic relationship but it can also happen with friends and family. If it is a family member, you have lived with it your whole life, it may be harder to identify. Read on and see if you can recognise any behaviour. When you first meet an abusive friend or romantic partner, they seem fine, and then it starts. They ring you or see you every day and they want to know what you are doing all of the time. A lot of them will shower you with gifts, flowers or they may just help out around your house. At first this is flattering and it makes you feel good as they seem really interested, however as time goes on you start to feel suffocated. All the attention can seem to be overwhelming and you may even try to end it. However the abusive one will bring you flowers or some other gift and will make you feel guilty and so you get back with them.

As time goes on the abusive/ controlling one will manipulate you so that all of your free time is spent with them. They will never tell you that you are not allowed to go out and that you have to stay with them. However they may say that they get upset that you go out without them while they are at work. They may make it difficult for you to go out with your friends by causing arguments. Eventually you just do not go out at all with your friends. They may tell you that they are lonely sitting at home while you go out having fun. The main point is that the abusive/ controlling one isolates you from your friends and family so that you spend most of your time with them. This happens gradually and a lot of the time you do not even notice that they are isolating you.

The abusive one will eventually become verbally, emotionally or physically abusive. However, some women may not even realise it especially if they are not being physically abused. If you are hit by the person, then you know that you need to leave the relationship. Whether you do leave or not is entirely up to you. However if you are being verbally or emotionally abused then there are no physical scars, so it is hard for you to realise that you are in an abusive relationship.

The abusive one also alters from being a kind and loving person to an angry one. A lot of the time you are left confused and you like to believe that the loving side is the 'real' person, that the angry side is just a bad mood and most people are moody aren't they? Wrong, there is a bad mood and then there is abuse. *The main tell-tale sign that you are in an abusive relationship is that you can be 'scared' of that person. In a 'healthy' romantic relationship you should never ever be scared of your partner, even during an argument.*

If you are feeling low, look at your relationship with your partner and see how the person makes you feel. If you realise that the person in your life is 'scary' sometimes and abusive then you have to decide if you are willing to fight for your happiness and leave. In this type of relationship there is no reduction of time with that person. The abusive one wants all of your spare time, so you need to end the relationship with this type of person.

There are many counsellors, psychologists, government organisations and women centres available that will be able to help you leave this type of person. Helplines are free and you can call them anonymously and get advice on what you need to do to leave your situation. Do not feel embarrassed to ask for help. Remember there are many people who have been in similar situations and have needed help to get out of them. That is why there is so much assistance out there. The main decision you have to make is that you are willing to fight for your freedom to be joyful and feel safe! That will mean ending a relationship that is harmful to you.

If you have children, then you can use your love for your children to give you the strength to leave an abusive relationship. Remember you have been blessed with children and you need to do everything in your power to ensure that they are safe. Watching violence in the home is just as harmful to children as being physically hit. Children are traumatised by watching their mother being abused and it affects their physical learning and development. If you cannot get out of your abusive situation for yourself, then use the love you have for your children to find your strength. Many women have been able to leave their violent partners because they want to protect their children. So use your love to gain the strength and courage to break away from a partner who may be verbally, emotionally and sometimes physically abusive. Yes you may love him despite the abuse but this is not about whether or not you love him. It is about you and your children's safety.

Boys who watch their mothers being beaten have a high likelihood of growing up and hitting their partners. While girls have a high likelihood of meeting men who are similar to their mother's abusers. They have grown up in an abusive environment so the behaviour from their abusive partners will appear to be 'normal' to them. You want the best for your children, so ask for help when you are ready to leave your partner. The cycle of abuse can be broken, but it is totally up to you.

Janet was married to Carl and she had two great kids Amy, aged five and Jack, aged three. After being married for five years, Janet realised that she was miserable in her relationship with her husband. They had their good days and their bad days but she was starting to feel very depressed.

So she went to a counsellor and explained her situation. Janet had thought that she was the problem, as nothing she did was good enough for her husband. All he seemed to do was criticise her and put down her appearance and tell her how bad she looked. If they went out and she drove, he would yell and tell her how she could not drive properly. Every meal she cooked had something wrong with it, and when she cleaned the house, there was always something that she did not do properly. Every time Janet did the 'wrong thing', Carl would get angry and yell at her. It got to the point that

Janet was walking on egg shells, as she never knew what mood he might be in or what she might do wrong that would make him angry. Unfortunately, she was not the only target as Carl would also yell at the children for doing "wrong things". Each day Janet and her children would wait to see what type of mood Carl was in, before they could decide how they would behave. Janet and the kids lived in fear daily as they were terrified of Carl getting angry with them.

After listening to Janet, the counsellor explained to Janet that she was living in domestic violence. Janet was shocked as she had thought that domestic violence was when the husband physically hit the wife. Carl had never hit Janet but when he got angry she was always fearful that one day he might actually hit her. The counsellor explained to Janet that she was experiencing verbal abuse from her husband, which was domestic violence. Janet felt lost and did not know what to do. So the counsellor gave her the name of a women's centre which would help Janet deal with her husband. A few weeks later, she took her children and left Carl. One year later Janet was happier than she had been in years. Carl was still giving her trouble but at least now she could make her own decisions and take control of her own life.

If you have a friend or family member whom you suspect is living in domestic violence then all you can do is offer your support. Try not to criticise their partners as this will only push them closer to their partners. Instead just tell them that you are there if they need any help. If they have children, then make them aware that they are harming their children by staying in the abusive relationship. Also realise that these women are adults and at the end of the day you cannot stop them from returning to their abusive partners. So try not to be too hard on yourself and just be there for them if they need you.

The fake

The fake is a person who basically talks about you behind your back. To your face they are nice and sweet, however when you are not around they are divulging everything about you to other friends. They also make negative comments about you to other people. You usually find out about the fake person because someone tells you about what they have said about you. Remember, if you notice people always saying negative things about other people when they are not around, then they are probably talking about you behind your back. Once again it is up to you if you want to associate with these types of "friends".

There are many different types of relationships which can make you feel low. Once you have identified who is making you feel this way, you have to decide how you want to deal with them. There are many options so you have to find one that will work for you and the other person (or people).

Yourself

Sometimes your own worst enemy is yourself as you are judgemental or feel guilty towards others and even more critical towards ourselves. A lot of us have grown up in families where guilt and judgement are seen as 'normal' behaviours. We see our parents having conversations where they talk about other people. For instance, you may have found out that a person you know is having an affair with a married man, and you are ready to label them both as bad people. The affair is between the people involved and has nothing to do with you. How would you feel if you were the person being judged? Does it hurt you to think that other people are talking about you? So why would you do it to others?

Wendy was shocked when she found out that her sister Amy was having an affair, as she believed that Amy was not the type of woman who went out with married men. A few years later, Wendy was going through her divorce and started dating

Scott at her work place. Scott had told Wendy that he was separated and it was only after a few weeks of dating, that Wendy found out that he was in fact still married and living with his wife and children. However, by this stage Wendy had fallen for him so she could not break off the relationship straight away. She continued to see him for a year before finally ending the relationship. The whole time Wendy was seeing Scott, she felt guilty and realised that she was wrong to judge her sister. Wendy did not think of herself as "that type" of woman and yet she was seeing a married man. She never knew the circumstances that led to her sister's affair and even if she did, it was not her business to criticise Amy. After a year of seeing Scott, Wendy eventually found out that he was having affairs with other women while he was seeing her. So she ended it with him and made sure she never judged anyone again.

We are our own worst critics and we need to be nicer to ourselves and those around us before we can be happier. So starting today, make a conscious effort to be kind and good to yourself and others. It is hard to be happy when you keep putting yourself down. So when anything happens in the future just observe and let it go. It is similar to noticing how your heart beats. Do you make a judgement about how fast or slow it beats? The answer is probably no, unless you are a doctor. So the next time you hear that Rita is having an affair with Tom, just acknowledge the information and then move onto another topic. I wonder who will win the Grand Final?

Coping with separation or divorce

If you decide that there is no way you are going to save your relationship and that you are ready to divorce or separate from your partner, then there are a few things you need to think about. No one ever talks to you about divorce, so a lot of you will find that it is probably one of the worst periods of your life. As I mentioned earlier, everyone is always talking about meeting a partner and the wedding. No one mentions the stress and the heart ache involved in a separation or divorce.

Before you even decide to go down this path, sit down and think if you have made the right decision. Is your relationship that unbearable that you need to break up? If you know you are living in domestic violence and are scared of your partner, then the answer is yes, it is time to leave. However, if domestic violence is not involved, then talk to your partner and see if the both of you can work it out. Perhaps see a counsellor and get them to help you with your relationship. There was a reason the two of you got married and hopefully counselling will help you rekindle what has been lost. After all the soul searching and counselling, you still decide to get divorced, then here are some ways of coping with what is about to happen to you.

When you go through a divorce, you are unable to think rationally. Your mind is confused as you are overwhelmed by feelings of anger, sadness, guilt and even shock depending on who ended the relationship. So the main thing you need to do is get yourself a diary and write everything down. There are many things that need to be sorted when you get divorced and a diary will help you think about what you need to do.

Firstly, try and see if you can negotiate with your ex-partner about the children and your assets. Family members may also be helpful in negotiating but only if they had a good relationship with your now ex-partner. However, if you are too overwhelmed, then go and see a lawyer as a last resort.

When you do select a lawyer, choose someone who has been recommended by a person you know or known through a friend.

Always listen to your gut instinct when selecting one. This is the time when you are most vulnerable and unfortunately there are a lot of people out there who like to prey on people who are going through a bad time and not thinking properly.

Your first session should normally be free (check with the receptionist when you make your appointment) and if you get a bad feeling or an uneasy feeling about the lawyer, then do not hire them. Lawyers are important and you have to select someone who will do the right thing by you. *This goes for everyone that you will meet while you are going through your divorce.* DO NOT SIGN ANYTHING straight away. Give yourself 24 hours to think about it before you sign up with any lawyer. If you find they are pressuring you, then move on and look for another lawyer. You should never feel pressured to sign anything. It would also help to have a support person with you when you see your lawyer, so they can step in if you find the meeting too much to handle.

If you do have children, remember that they will be upset by the break up, so organise some counselling for them, even if it is only for a few sessions. You may find that seeing a counsellor is helpful to you too. Remember they are only there to give you counselling support, not financial or legal matters. Once again listen to your gut instinct, if the counsellor wants you to do something that makes your stomach churn and makes you feel uncomfortable then leave! Find someone else whom you can feel at ease with.

The division of the family assets can be peaceful if both partners trust each other. However, make sure you get your own independent legal advice before signing anything prepared by your partner's solicitor. The chapter on finances will give you a better understanding about money and how you can get a better grasp on your own finances.

Making yourself happy by being surrounded by positive people

So the next time you feel low and reach for that chocolate bar or credit card, stop for a minute and look at whom or what is making you feel that way. Once you start to see a pattern, you can decide how you want to deal with them.

To make yourself happy, you may have to reduce contact with the people who are making you feel bad. This may mean not seeing some close family members or friends for a period of time. Once you feel you are able to cope with them again, you can resume contact but this time on your terms. That is, see them every few months as opposed to every weekend or even every day. It can be hard in the beginning but after a few weeks, when you notice how much better you feel, you will find that it will be easier to surround yourself with people who support you and make you feel good.

The law of attraction and attracting positive relationships into your life

The saying goes when one door closes another opens. So while you may find that some of your negative relationships may come to an end, new ones will begin as you start life afresh. As explained earlier the law of attraction simply states that like attracts like. So if you are happy then you will attract positive people and circumstances. Alternatively, if you are angry and depressed you are going to attract angry and depressed people and circumstances. With this in mind the next section will look at how you can use the law of attraction to bring positive people and situations into your life.

Many individuals are finding that they are actually satisfied being single and are only interested in having platonic friendships in their lives. Others are looking for their romantic life partner. The next section can help you find both.

Saying Thank You

The first thing to do is to be thankful for what you do have. To attract positive relationships you need to be positive and appreciative for what you already have in your life.

At this point you may be thinking yeah right, but I still have to go to that job I hate, or look after my toddler that is crying. Let me put it in perspective for you. Do you think that everyone in the world is as lucky as you are? What about the millions of starving people in Africa? When they get up every morning, what do they think? Do the mothers wonder if they are able to feed their children? Whether they will be able to live another day?

I am not trying to trivialise your problems, I want you to realise how blessed you are to be able to sit and read this book. Not everyone in the world has this opportunity and you need to be thankful for the simple things that you do have in your life now.

So as you go through your day, find little things to be thankful for and even people to say thank you to. Some more examples of being thankful for are:

- Thank you for my beautiful children
- Thank you for my great partner
- Thank you for my car
- Thank you for my job
- Thanks you for my healthy body

Affirmations or mantras

Affirmations or mantras are positive phrases that you repeat, so that you can start to change the way you think. When we are depressed our brain thinks in a certain way. During the day, just sit back and listen to what you are thinking, I mean really listen. Are the thoughts in your head positive or negative? What is it saying about your relationships? What is your mind thinking when you are talking to the people in your life? Do the thoughts make you feel energised or depressed?

Feeling low alters the way you view the world. For instance, when you are low, do you notice the beautiful sunny day outside or are you too absorbed in your problems to notice everything around you. You would drive or catch the train to work, all the while thinking about all the issues in your life. When you dwell on your troubles you become sadder and create more issues. A lot of people believe that they will be happy once their problems have disappeared. This is incorrect. In fact, you need to start LIVING now and enjoying life NOW. Once you start to have a positive outlook, you will see your troubles will lessen. The problems in your life relate to how you view them. If you change the way you look at them, you can reduce the way they affect your life.

Sally was going to a fancy dress party and she needed to find a dress that would suit her. Every weekend she went out shopping looking for the perfect outfit, however she could not find the right dress. She was getting depressed and it was all she could think about.

One lunch time she was talking to Lily at work about her problem, when Kate walked up to them. "Sorry to interrupt" she said but I overheard your conversation about the dress. There is a warehouse in Richmond which has really good costumes. I think they have a sale at the moment and you may be able to get an outfit for a real bargain."

"Oh thanks so much Kate. I will have a look tomorrow during my lunch break," replied Sally.

The next day Sally went to the warehouse and found the perfect dress for her party. She was overjoyed as she came back to work. Sally went to Kate's desk to thank her and found that she was not there. The next day Sally went looking for Kate and still could not find her, so she went to see her Kate's boss. "Excuse me Greg, do you know if Kate is in today".

"Kate is in hospital" replied Greg. "Her son's leukaemia is getting worse and he was readmitted."

Sally stood staring at Greg in shock. Here she was complaining about her dress and she had never heard Kate complaining about her son. Suddenly the problem with her dress seemed so trivial and she realised that not finding the right dress was not a problem after all. From that day onwards Sally stopped stressing over the little things in life and appreciated the fact that she and her family were healthy.

Once you have changed the way you look at the problems in your life, you can start to say affirmations and change the way you think. This will help you to make changes in your life now.

At first this may all sound a bit farfetched and ridiculous, but if you are feeling down, have you got anything to lose by trying these new strategies? The worst that can happen is that you remain the way you are, while the best thing that can happen is that your life actually starts to change and you become happier. Decide if you want to follow these strategies and change your life for the better.

The following are some examples of affirmations that you can say to yourself whenever you remember. You can write them all down and say them every morning when you get up and at night when you go to bed. These affirmations can be placed around your home so that you will read them throughout your day.

I have loving and happy relationships in my life.
My family and I are happy.
My family and I are divinely protected.

I have positive relationships in my life.
I have positive relationships at work.
I have loving and supportive relationships in my life.
I have a loving and caring partner.

Attracting Your Partner and other positive people

Many women believe that they will be happy once they meet their Prince Charming. Unfortunately this is not the case and too many women get married, find that they are still unhappy and then separate or get divorced. Before you meet Mr Right, you have to feel positive within yourself. If you are happy within yourself, then according to the law of attraction you are going to attract a partner who is also happy. If you are depressed and angry, then you are going to attract people who are sad and hostile and will make you unhappy. Only you have the power to make yourself be happy.

Always remember though that you do not need a partner to feel complete or blissful. You can be satisfied being by yourself and doing the things that interest you. Too many women feel that they need to have a man in their life, but this is not the case and in today's society we can be joyful, strong, independent single women.

At one of my work places there was a woman named Maria who was about thirty years old. She was from Spain and had originally moved to Australia to study and then started working. Maria was one of the happiest women I had ever met. When I questioned her about why she did not have a boyfriend, she said that she did not need to have a partner. Maria enjoyed living by herself and doing things that made her happy. She had her work, friends and life was relaxed and fun. I am unsure if this was unique to Maria's family or whether it was a Spanish philosophy. However after watching Maria, I started to see that it was OK being single, and that my life was blissful. Maria's carefree attitude rubbed off on me, as I started to see that we have been fortunate enough to be living in a great country and time, when women are able to lead fulfilling single lives.

If you find that you are jumping from one unhappy relationship to another, you need to spend some time by yourself. You may be surprised at how you may actually enjoy your own company.

I struggled with my unhappiness for many years and during that time I attracted people and circumstances that made me even more depressed. Sometimes it is hard to be positive when bad things have happened in your life, such as a difficult childhood. However, you need to give yourself a time period to get over the unpleasant events and then you need to start doing things that make you happy now. What happened to you was in the past and you cannot change it. ***You can only find happiness when you realise that you have to give up ever hoping for a better past.*** You need to focus on the now and creating a contented life.

To find what makes YOU smile is totally up to you. Everyone is different and you need to find out what makes you light up on the inside. When I found myself single again, I decided to do things that I had always wanted to do but just never had the time. I started writing and getting back into my drawing and painting. These were activities which I enjoyed but just never had the time to do, as I was busy working, raising my children and being in relationships. Suddenly when I was single again and had time when the children went to visit their dad, I decided to do the things which made me happy.

Your idea of happiness might be going hiking, cooking or simply watching movies. If it makes you happy and it does not hurt anyone else, then do it. Once you are smiling more often, you will find that you will start to attract nicer people, including a partner that is both supportive and loving.

You may wonder why I keep emphasising happiness and the answer is simple. For years I tried to be happy through romantic relationships. Now I am truly the happiest that I have ever been, and I want to share it with everyone else. I want you to know that you do not have to be living in fear, depression and anger. I did that for many years and did not believe that I could change. Now that I am enjoying life and my freedom, there is no way that I could compromise my lifestyle.

Listen to your gut instinct when meeting people

This is an especially important concept and everyone needs to listen to your gut instinct or inner voice. When you first meet someone you usually have some type of reaction to them. It may be that you like them instantly and you feel as though you have known them forever. Alternatively, you may get a bad feeling about them and your stomach starts to churn. When you get this bad feeling about someone, you need to listen to your gut instinct and have little or nothing to do with them. Then there are others who are just neutral and you do not have any real strong reaction to them initially. However, as you get to know them, something in your mind tells you to stay away from them. Listen to that voice! Your gut instinct is your warning sign to what you cannot see about that person. Remember your gut instinct and the little voice in your head, knows what it is talking about. You can probably look back and think how your first impressions about a certain person were correct.

A friend of mine named Judith, who had two girls named Shelly and Crystal, was going through a very rough divorce with her ex-husband. Judith was dating someone but that relationship ended. She had met him through online dating, so she decided to get back online and meet someone new. After being on line for a few weeks, she struck a connection with Paul and after a few emails and phone calls; she decided to meet him for lunch. Judith picked a café she knew so that she could feel safe. When Judith first met Paul, she did not have a strong reaction. He was dressed a bit too casual, which was something Judith had never really liked. However, Judith sat down and had lunch with him. After lunch they stepped out of the restaurant and Paul immediately asked Judith on a second date. Judith agreed and they realised that the only time that they could meet was when he had his three year old daughter. Judith loved children so she agreed to go to his place on the Friday and he would cook them dinner. Paul then started to text Judith every day, stating that he was attracted to her because she was such a spiritual person. A few days later, Judith went to Paul's place and she met his beautiful daughter who looked like Shirley Temple with her curly blonde hair and large blue eyes. They ate dinner, put his daughter to bed and then sat on the couch to have a chat. As they talked, Paul mentioned some strange topics and all of a sudden a little voice in Judith's head told her to leave the house. Judith ignored her gut instinct and reasoned with herself that Paul could not be bad as he was looking after his daughter. She was cute and adorable and surely if Paul was a bad person, his ex-wife would not let him look after their daughter. So Judith ignored her inner voice and stayed with Paul.

A few weeks later she noticed that he would disappear outside a few times a day and she realised that he had lied about being a non-smoker on his online dating profile. However, Judith decided to overlook the fact that Paul had lied to her. She thought that the fact that he was so helpful around the house and was always going out of his way to help her, made up for the lie about smoking.

Months passed by quickly and Judith was starting to feel suffocated by Paul. She eventually told him that she wanted to end the relationship. Paul started crying and when Judith saw the tears in his eyes, she felt sorry for him. He looked devastated and she did not have the heart to leave.

Their relationship developed quickly and within a year, Paul had moved into Judith's house with his daughter. Time went on and everything seemed to be going well. There was another occasion when Judith's inner voice, told her to leave, but once again she ignored her gut instinct. Whenever they had a fight and Judith spoke about leaving, Paul would cry and even talk about committing suicide. So Judith felt sorry for Paul and she kept working at the relationship.

Judith began having unsettling feelings about Paul, so she questioned her daughters to make sure that everything was alright. She never came out and asked her daughters if Paul was molesting them but encouraged them to talk to her if anything happened. Both her daughters told her that life was fine.

Time went on and Judith and Paul started making plans for their future together. Then one day, Judith's older daughter named Shelley came to Judith and told her that Paul had touched her inappropriately. Judith was shocked and when she confronted Paul, he denied it. He stated that Shelley had made it up as she was jealous of their relationship and of Paul being in their lives. Paul was pretty convincing but Judith also knew her daughter. Shelley would not have made up something like that. Judith kicked Paul out of her house and was left feeling shocked and angry. How could she have exposed her children to such danger? Judith took Shelley to a counsellor and reported Paul to the police. During counselling Judith learned that children (even teenage girls) sometimes keep quiet because they do not want the abuser hurting their mother or siblings. They also want to make their mother happy and revealing anything bad about their abuser might upset their mother.

It is up to mothers and fathers to look after their children. If you feel uneasy about any particular person being around your children, then you need to stop that person having contact with them. Children are innocent and do not have the skills to always tell you when something is wrong. It might be an idea to also teach your children about listening to their gut instinct.

Looking back Judith recalled her inner voice and how she had ignored it. It was a tough lesson for her but one that she will always remember. She allowed me to retell her story to you, so that other women could learn from her experience. Bad people do not always look bad, so our gut instinct lets us know what we cannot see, that is their bad character. You might be going through a tough time in your life but your gut instinct will always help you work out what people are like.

Remember that some of the worst criminals are also the most charming and manipulative. They know what to say and how to say it, to get you to do what they want.

Jacob told me a story about a time when he was a young man and he lost all his money to a 'friend'. When he was 18 years old he shared a house with four other young men. One of them named Laurie told the others that they could double their money if they placed a bet on a particular horse. Laurie was a charming young man and all the boys thought he was great. They all liked and trusted Laurie and gave him all their savings. He took their money and disappeared. The young men were devastated by the loss of their money and trust. They had however learned a valuable lesson that people who are untrustworthy can be charming.

Your list

When you are ready to meet your new partner or friends, you need to think about the type of person you do want in your life. This is important, as you need to ignore what you do not want. For instance, Judith had been concerned about meeting a man who might abuse her children and she had attracted Paul into her life. You need to only focus on what you want in your partner.

Mary, a friend of mine, was an attractive, professional and intelligent woman. She had paid to join various dating agencies; however she was not having any luck. Mary was getting quite disheartened as she could not find a man that would commit to her. So over a coffee I told her to make a list of her perfect partner.

"But I'm really picky" said Mary "That's fine." I replied "Just write down exactly what you want in a guy".

"Ok, I'll give it a go" declared Mary.

Now Mary had read the same books that I had including the one that I had been recommended by my two friends. However, Mary did not find the books useful. I did however expect her to have a basic understanding of the law of attraction, so it surprised me when I received the following e-mail from her, later that day.

Hi Karen,

I did up a list of preferences for what I'm looking for in a man. What do you think? I might add to it after Sunday's date.

Mary

The List
   Not an ocker!!!!!!!!!! Very important
   Outgoing
   Even temperament
   Not commitment phobic

Co-ordinated—can play tennis, squash and other
racket sports
Not materialistic
Honest
Reliable
Tactful
Height: 5'7 and above
Articulate
Respects and likes women
Has a good sense of humour
Enjoys social interaction with friends
Not possessive or jealous
Retains own sense of identity—does not have to
be with partner 24/7
What you see is what you get. Not a total psycho
behind closed doors
Has a good relationship with family
Values and interests align with my own
Strong personality but not controlling
Good interpersonal skills
Awareness of current affairs
Not manipulative
Considerate
Good posture
Good eating habits
Earns enough to be able to save some money

After reading her e-mail I gave her the following advice.

Hi Mary,

The first thing is to focus on what you want, not on what you do not want. If it is on your list then you will attract that type of guy. Have you noticed that you are meeting ockers? (By the way, ockers are basically men who are a bit rough around the edges, loud and like to drink a lot.) So don't even have the word ocker on your list.

Don't write not commitment phobic as you will attract men who are.

Don't write "not materialistic" as you will attract materialistic men.

Don't write "Not jealous or possessive" as you will attract jealous and possessive men. Basically only write down what you want. Don't even mention what you don't want.

So your list might be:
    Outgoing
    Even temperament
    Ready for commitment
    Coordinated—can play tennis, squash and other
        racket sports

Honest
Reliable
Tactful
Height: 5'7 and above
Articulate
Respects and likes women
Has a good sense of humour
Enjoys social interaction with friends
Retains own sense of identity
Independent
Easy going
Caring
Has a good relationship with family
Values and interests align with my own
Strong personality
Good interpersonal skills
Awareness of current affairs
Considerate
Good posture
Good eating habits
Good at budgeting his money

What do you think?

Karen.

Mary eventually wrote back to tell me that what I said made sense, especially when she looked at the men she had dated in the past.

So when you are feeling positive within yourself, and are ready to date, you need to make a list of the type of person you want in your life. ***Just remember that you might unconsciously think of things that you do not want in a partner, but your gut instinct will help you realise this, so that you can move on and find Mr Right.***

Vision Board or Dream Board

An additional way, to attract a partner is to have a "vision" or "dream" board. This is taking a piece of cardboard or a pin board and putting pictures of the type of man you want in your life. You can also write down the characteristics that you want to attract and have them pinned or stuck onto your vision board. As I mentioned earlier, do not dismiss it until you try it. Start with something small and write down what you want and have a picture of it on your vision board. Then sit back and see what happens. It also helps to have a date of when you expect to have it. Remember whatever you ask for has to be achievable for you. There is no point putting a million dollars on your vision board if you do not believe it is going to happen.

Believing you have it now

This step is essential as in order for you to manifest what you want, that is, you need to believe that you will have it. It requires a bit of imagination, as you pretend that you are going to meet your perfect partner. Have fun with this and believe that they are entering your life soon. This may all sound fanciful but just try it and see what happens. If you are ready to meet Mr Right and you have nothing better to do then try these strategies and see what happens.

The New Improved You

When looking at improving your life you have to make a pact with yourself to do everything in your power to make you happy now! Not tomorrow, not in a weeks' time, and especially not in the New Year (unless today is the New Year). You have to start today by making little changes. This may be acknowledging what happened in your past has already happened and that you cannot change it.

You have to stop thinking about the past and wishing that your life had turned out differently. Move on and focus on the here and now and make every effort to fight for your happiness. A lot of us keep replaying our past in our minds, again and again and again. This is not productive and will leave you stuck in the past. You have to make a conscious effort to stop thinking about it and enjoy what is happening now. The future has not happened yet and you can make a difference.

Too many of us also put ourselves last and focus on our family and friends first, which then causes everyone else to put you last as well. You have to realise that you are worth it and you deserve to be living in bliss. When you are feeling good and wake up excited every morning, you will find that you will attract positive people and events and your whole life will change for the better.

Chapter 3

Losing Weight

Most women today seem to be unhappy with their bodies and are trying to lose weight. They have probably been on at least one diet in their life. Diets do not help you lose weight. In fact thinking about losing weight, does not help you lose weight. To reduce your weight to a level that makes you happy involves a number of strategies. Just following one of the steps below will not work. You need to follow all the steps in order to reach your ideal weight.

When you are born you are happy with your body. You do not lie in your cot thinking "This nappy makes my bum look big". Life is interesting and you are too immersed in what is going on around you to pay any attention to your body. That is the way you need to start to think about your body. You need to believe that you are naturally slim and focus on enjoying your life. Thinking about losing weight takes up a lot of your energy, so that you do not enjoy the wonderful things that life has to offer.

When you start to believe that you are slim, you will see exactly how great life is and be amazed at how your weight will just drop off. Naturally slim people do not even think about losing weight. You need to think like a naturally slim person who has never worried about their weight in their life. The following strategies will help you get to this stage.

Step 1—Making positive changes to your life

The first thing you need to do is find out how to make yourself be more positive. When you have issues with weight, there is something in your life that is upsetting you. Your reason for feeling empty or in pain is not always so obvious, especially when you have a busy life trying to juggle everything around you. The main thing to remember is that those surrounding you should treat you with respect, kindness and non-judgement. More importantly you have to allow your inner thoughts to be supportive and encouraging.

The chapters on "Relationship with you" will help you work on yourself and help you to value and appreciate yourself. Too many of you have put your own needs and wants aside to care for others. The chapter on relationships will help you look after your spirit so that you can be happier within yourself. At the very least, it will help you realise that you need to take care of yourself first before you can really help anyone else.

The chapter on "Relationships" has tools to help you identify any relationships in your life which you need to work on. Most of the time you are so involved and busy in your day to day life, that you do not even realise how unhealthy your relationships with other people in your life may be. Once you realise which ones are not working, you can then try and see if you can resolve the issues yourself or seek help from a trusted professional counsellor. Just remember we all deserve to be treated with respect, kindness and non-judgement from all our family and friends. If they truly love and care for you, they will ensure that they come to a compromise to make you happy. However if they continue to treat you with disrespect then you have to look at the options of either reducing contact with them or removing them from your life. You will find that once you remove people who make you feel dreadful, then you will meet more positive people.

There are other reasons which may cause you to be overweight. Sometimes there are so many issues in your life that you are unable to narrow down just one reason. However the main way to track down the actual cause of your weight gain is to look around the time you started to put on weight.

What happened in your life to suddenly make you feel troubled and gain weight? This will require you to pause, take a step back and try and identify what was the cause for the extra inches. Once you can narrow down the 'trigger' for your weight gain, you can then get some professional counselling on how to cope with the negative feelings from that experience.

Chantelle was overweight and she had tried to lose weight by herself without any success, so she tried hypnotherapy with a psychologist. At her first appointment, Chantelle discussed her past history and mentioned that she had a miscarriage a couple of months earlier. Chantelle also had an abusive childhood and had stopped having contact with her parents. The psychologist tried to hypnotise Chantelle to lose weight and during the session they talked about what type of diet Chantelle needed to follow. Six sessions later, Chantelle had not lost any weight and she still felt depressed, so she stopped seeing the psychologist.

A few months later, Chantelle fell pregnant and had a healthy baby. Six months after the birth of her baby, Chantelle lost her weight without any problem. She was back to her weight prior to her miscarriage. Chantelle then realised that the psychologist should have treated her for depression, not weight loss. She was grieving and had not made the connection with her weight gain. It was only after she had stopped grieving was she able to lose her weight easily.

Sometimes when you do see a professional they are trying to treat the "weight" problem when the increased inches is just a symptom of some other experience which is making you unhappy. Take a few deep breaths and look at your life. Think about what has happened that has caused you to gain the weight? This may be over a long period of time or over a short period.

Here is a list of possible experiences which may cause you to feel bad and put on weight:

- Childhood abuse
- Growing up in a home with domestic violence
- Neglected childhood
- Miscarriage
- Relationship break up
- Death of a friend, family member or pet
- Bullying
- Sexual assault /rape
- Relationship with domestic violence
- Relationship where you felt your partner neglected you
- Low self esteem

This list is not exhaustive, but I hope it gives you an idea of the events that may have happened in your past which caused you to gain weight.

Most of you may have tried to deal with the situation yourself or just ignored it. You may even believe that you have recovered from the event. However, if you are still unable to lose weight then chances are you have not recovered from it and you need to talk to someone. In all these cases it may be helpful to see a counsellor whom you can trust to help you. Sessions with an expert may help close the chapter of your past and allow you to focus on what is happening now and in the future.

Step 2—Focus on being healthy— Stop trying to lose weight

Starting today, you are to stop trying to lose weight. No, this is not a typo. Instead focus on being 'healthy' and this will help you take your mind off food and the whole idea about 'losing weight'. The more you focus on your eating issues and keep thinking that you want to stop eating, the worse it will get.

By focusing on something else, you will eventually forget that you even have any weight issues. It may take a while to work but the first step is to forget about your eating habits and focus on just being 'healthy'.

What do you think naturally skinny or slim people think about? Do you think they are sitting there thinking about losing weight? The answer is no. They are busy with their day to day lives and are not even giving a second thought to losing weight. Their main focus is on being healthy and enjoying what life has to offer. So starting today, focus on having a healthy body now and believe that you are naturally slim.

Step 3—Change your mindset and believe that you are naturally slim

What are you saying to yourself about your body? Start paying attention to the thoughts in your mind. Are you telling yourself that you are fat? Is your mind telling you that you are naturally overweight? Is it telling you that your family are all large so you are too? It's just genetics? When you do lose weight, are you thinking "The weight will come back again, it always does", "I just can't lose weight no matter how hard I try". "I have always been overweight, so the weight will come back."

Listen carefully to your mind, what is it saying? If you believe that you are naturally fat then you will spend your whole life focused on trying to lose weight. *So starting today, believe that you are naturally slim. Your aim now is to be healthy and forget about weight loss.*

Stop having negative thoughts about your body and just believe that you are perfect just the way you are. Whenever you do have a critical thought about your body, swap it straightaway with a positive thought such as "I am naturally slim".

This thought is called an affirmation and it will help you change the way you think about your body.

Step 4—Daily affirmations or mantras

Affirmations or mantras help you change the way you think so that you will believe that you are naturally slim and healthy.

When you say affirmations, you are changing years of critical self-talk about yourself. I realised just how powerful affirmations were when I started to say them every day. You can test how well they work by saying them daily. Remember you have been thinking a certain way up until now. Let us say you are twenty years old, so for the past five years you may have had certain negative beliefs about your body and your weight. It will take you some time to change the way you think, so keep working at it and over time it will happen.

Say or think your affirmations as many times as you remember. When you are driving to work, catching the train, or even when you are having a shower. The more often you say them during the day, the more they will work.

Samantha heard about affirmations so she decided to see if they worked. She decided to think "I am slim and beautiful" and would think of her daily positive statements whenever she remembered. If she started to criticise herself with a comment such as "My hips are big", she replaced it straight away with "I am naturally slim". A few months later, she found that people were describing her using the words in her affirmations and she was changing to suit her statements.

She had been saying to herself "I am slim and attractive" and after a few months, people started complementing her and telling her that she was attractive. Sam was not doing anything else differently, but she noticed that she started to feel better about her own body image. She also noticed that she started to crave healthier foods such as fruit and vegetables, whereas previously she used to snack on chocolate and biscuits. She still occasionally reached for a chocolate bar but she did not beat herself up about it. Since she stopped denying herself foods such as chocolate, she automatically ate everything in moderation. Samantha realised that all food was okay to eat. Her biggest discovery was that she also started to accept her own body and this change in mindset showed her the power of affirmations.

Some positive statements that you may like to say are:

I am beautiful
I have beautiful hair, eyes, feet etc
I have a healthy body
I am naturally slim

These are only a few and you can make up your own. Just remember to say it as though you already have it and believe that it is true in your heart.

At first the affirmations may seem untrue, but after saying it for a while you will start to believe it and you will start to see the changes taking place in your life. This will reinforce what you are saying to yourself. Like Sam, I used to think that I was naturally overweight but now I think that I am naturally slim. You can do this too, you just have to believe in yourself.

Step 5—Visualisation

When you close your eyes and see yourself in your mind, what do you physically look like? How would you describe yourself? If you have issues with your weight and eating, then chances are that you see yourself in a negative way in your mind. You need to change what you believe you look like into what you want to actually look like.

First close your eyes and see yourself as a slim person. If you find it hard to see yourself in this way, find a picture of yourself when you were at your ideal weight, if you have one. Alternatively think of a person who has the body that you like and then replace their face, with yours. Take your time, do not rush, just breathe and let it happen.

Do not give up and everyday keep trying until you can see yourself as a slim and healthy person in your mind. When you think of yourself from now on, see the naturally slim person you were born to be.

Step 6—Regular Exercise

Exercise is not something you do to lose weight. The main reason you need to exercise is to remain healthy and feel good. When you exercise your body releases endorphins which is a naturally feel good chemical. It also reduces stress so that you are left feeling happier and more positive about your life.

Physical activity does not have to be anything too hard and it does not have to cost you anything. The best way to start is to just go for a walk. You can do it anywhere, for instance, you can go for a quick walk during your lunch break. If you have not exercised in a while, start small, and then work your way up. Eventually you will be doing at least thirty minutes of exercise a day.

Walking is a great way to clear your mind and increase your positive energy. I have always found that walking makes me feel good. There is a treadmill at my home so that I can exercise any time of the day and in all kinds of weather. When you are feeling a bit down, a brisk walk will actually start to lift your spirit.

Once again, you do not have to take my word for it. Put on your shoes and go for a walk and see how you feel afterwards. Chances are you will be better.

Any form of exercise is good, so if you do not like walking then try something else. There are plenty to choose from, and the key is to find an activity that you enjoy so that you will do it as part of your lifestyle. If you get bored doing the same thing day after day, then find a variety of exercises. The key is to keep trying until you find the right combination. There is no use going out and joining a gym if you know that you cannot do it forever. That is why I suggested something easy such as walking briskly which is easy, free and can be done anywhere and anytime.

Here is a list of the type of exercise that you could do:

- walking
- running/jogging
- dancing
- karate/martial arts

A friend of mine named Katie works long hours in a stressful job, so she hired a personal trainer to help motivate her to exercise. The session with the personal trainer encourages her each night to make her way to the gym, as she has already made an appointment with her trainer. Katie is the type of person who needs someone to push her to exercise and that is fine. You may be able to find a few friends who are interested in starting up a walking group. The main focus is to exercise to stay fit and feel good.

Step 7—Are you intolerant to certain foods?

Many of you may have been trying to lose weight and have found that you are not feeling 100%. Sometimes the reason you are not feeling good is because you have intolerances to different types of food.

Anastasia had always felt as though her stomach was bloated. She would exercise and do a hundred sit ups each day. However no matter how hard she tried, her stomach always felt uncomfortable and big. Anastasia had felt like this her whole life and just thought that she was one of those people who put weight on her stomach. When she eventually got married and had a baby, she developed dermatitis on her hands from constant hand washing. Anastasia tried countless medications and natural creams to cure the dermatitis. It would get better for a short period of time and then eventually return with full force. Anastasia was sick of having cracked and bleeding hands. She was also starting to have severe stomach problems and would feel tired and lethargic for most of the day.

Then one day she met Peter who suggested that she see a doctor who specialised in naturopathy. The doctor put Anastasia on an elimination diet and gave her a list of foods that she had to stop eating. He also gave her some natural supplements that she had to take every day. During the first few days of her diet she found that she was always hungry and irritable. She stuck to her diet and after a week she started to notice the difference. Anastasia's dermatitis was disappearing and she was feeling good. It was the first time in her life where her stomach did not feel bloated and uncomfortable. She felt so good, that it motivated her to stick to the elimination diet. In the next stage of the diet, Anastasia had to re-introduce one type of food each time to see if she reacted to it. If there was a bad reaction, then she had to stop eating it. She found that she reacted to dairy, gluten, oranges and tomato. Once Anastasia avoided those foods, she started to feel healthy and positive about her body.

If you do feel bloated most of the time or your body just does not feel right, then discuss it with your doctor. If you do not have a doctor, then ask your friends, work colleagues and family for one. It is amazing how help comes to you when you ask for it. So put your request out to the universe and help will come. Make sure you write down all your symptoms no matter how small you think they are. The more information you can give your doctor, the better they will be able to help you. Remember you deserve to feel good so put your health first.

Step 8—Stop dieting and eat well every couple of hours

Too many people go on diets or skip meals to lose weight. This does not work in the long term. You have probably experienced this yourself when you went on a diet, lost weight but put it all back on a few months later. So then you go back on another diet to lose weight, you lose the weight, then a few months later, guess what, you have put the weight back on. This clearly shows that diets do not help you lose weight in the long term.

First thing you will need to realise is that you need to make a lifestyle change. This means that whatever steps you take to lose weight now, you need to do for the rest of your life. It needs to be changes that you can live with forever. Everyone is different so the changes have to be easy and comfortable for you.

Too many young girls and women "diet" or starve themselves believing that they will lose weight. The problem with starving yourself is that it lowers your metabolism, so that food will be burned slowly by your body. Your body thinks it is in starvation mode so it actually tries to make the food last longer by using it up slowly. This is a survival mechanism in your body which has helped humans survive through famines.

When you stop your diet and start to eat regularly again, you will find that you will put on the weight you lost, plus more. This is because your body's metabolism has slowed down from your dieting. Your body is burning food at a slower rate and any extra food you are now eating will be stored as fat. The human body thinks that you might starve again, so it stores the food.

In order to show you what I mean by metabolism and food, here is an example of how our body works. Imagine you have a car and you use as much fuel as you need. Suddenly there is a world-wide fuel shortage so you can only use 3 litres of fuel a day. For three months, you use 3 litres of fuel a day and you get used to it. Then one day a new supply of fuel is found and you can have as much fuel as you want again. You still remember how tough it was to only survive on 3 litres of fuel a day, so you start to store some fuel in drums at home. Like fuel, your body remembers not having enough food and it stores the food as fat. To lose weight you need to stop dieting and keep your metabolism up by eating every couple of hours.

Farah was a naturally slim and attractive girl however she always felt as though she was overweight and ordinary. Friends and strangers would compliment Farah on her looks but the words had no meaning for her. Deep down inside Farah felt miserable about herself and nothing anyone else said or did could help her feel better. When Farah left school and started to work, she decided that she was going to go on a diet to lose weight. She also joined the gym and exercised seven days a week. Farah went from a slim girl to a very thin young woman. One year later Farah started to eat all the foods that she had denied herself. She found that she started to put on weight and was bigger than when she first started going to the gym. Dieting had actually caused Farah to put on weight in the long run.

Dieting or starving yourself is dangerous for your health and does not help you lose weight forever. The key to maintain a slim body is to eat moderate portions of food regularly, such as every few hours, and allow yourself any type of food.

Step 9—Eat whatever you want—there is no such thing as bad food

After you stop dieting you need to start eating moderately and believe that all food is the same. There are no bad foods and good foods. It is true that some foods are healthier for you than others, however you need to change your mind set to believe that all food is the same. This belief will remove any feelings of guilt you will have when you eat food such as chocolate. Too many people categorise certain foods like chocolate for example as bad foods, so they tell themselves that they are not allowed to eat it. The more you deny yourself something, the more you think about it and the more you want it. You just have to look at your own behaviours to see how true this is.

How many of you tell yourself that you are not allowed to have chocolate? The longer you deny yourself the chocolate, the more you think about it and the more you want it. When you do eventually eat the chocolate, you will probably eat too much and then feel guilty. To prevent this from happening, you need to believe that all food is the same and if you do feel like chocolate, allow yourself to have some. You will find that when you stop denying yourself certain foods, you will stop wanting to eat them.

Step 10—Stop comparing your body to others

Do not compare yourself to others and start to believe that you are perfect just the way you are.

How many of you have looked at magazines and compared yourselves to the beautiful models on their pages? Even watched a movie where the gorgeous actress on the screen made you feel bad about your own body. Comparing your body to other people's body is only going to make you unhappy. You need to realise that everyone is different and you have your own unique body shape.

Women have numerous body shapes and sizes and they are all different. When you compare yourself to a model for instance, it is like comparing your height with a model's height. There is no way you can grow anymore so that you are the same height as that model. The same goes for your body. There is no way you can diet so much that you will have exactly the same bum, stomach or legs as the model. You have to realise that your body is perfect just the way it is.

Magazines alter the images of the models, so that the pictures you are looking at do not really exist. It is like comparing yourself to a cartoon character. The original picture may have been the model but after digital enhancement you are left with an unrealistic image. By the end of the editing process, the original model does not look like the final picture when it appears in the magazine. It is all make believe and these women do not exist.

There are plenty of organisations who will be able to supply you with information on just how the beauty magazine industry alters their model's images. You would be amazed what technology can do.

You may wonder why the magazines do this, and the very simple answer is that they want to sell a product. When you see a gorgeous model using a certain brand of perfume and then next to her is this gorgeous male model, it sends you a message that if you buy that perfume you can be gorgeous and attract a hot guy. That is a very basic idea of the psychology that magazines use to encourage their readers to buy products.

The fact that the magazines have to alter the images, just shows you that even the models that you think are 'perfect' are not good enough for a magazine. Imagine how the models must feel when they see their own photos being changed so much that they cannot even recognise themselves. Chances are the models also have issues with their own bodies.

Comparing yourself to other people will only make you miserable, so accept your body just the way it is, and you will start to feel a lot more positive and at ease.

Step 11—Have a good night's sleep or nap during the day

It is very important that you sleep well, so that you are able to remain positive during the day. When you do not have enough sleep, you will find that you will get tired and moody. You will also eat and drink foods that you would not normally eat, just to get some energy during the day and feel better. These foods are usually high in sugar or caffeine and give you a quick boost of energy but will only make you feel worse later.

An adult requires approximately eight hours of sleep each night, while teenagers need a lot more sleep as their bodies are developing. Each of us is different and our bodies will need different hours of sleep. Pay attention to how you feel when you have various hours of sleep. You may need more or less, then the 8 hours. If you cannot sleep properly during the night, then try to have a nap during the middle of the day. Do not have a nap close to your bed time, as this may affect your sleep.

When you are stressed or worried about something, you may find that you are unable to sleep well. This is especially true when you are going through a relationship break up. You may suffer from insomnia, or keep waking up many times during the night. This is very frustrating as you lie awake and try to force yourself to sleep.

Some ways of helping you to sleep are:

- Get into a routine where you go to bed and wake up at the same time each day.
- If you are worried about something, have a diary by your bed where you can write down

everything that you are worried about. Once your thoughts are on paper, you may be able to forget about it while you are asleep. This is especially useful when you are going through a stressful time.

- Focus on having a good night's sleep. The last thing you want to say to yourself at night is "I hope I sleep tonight'. This is setting yourself up to fail, as you expect to not sleep properly at night. Stop worrying about it and just sleep. Repeat to yourself that you are going to have a good night's sleep.

- Meditate or do relaxation exercises just before you go to bed. Sitting in a quiet room and focusing on your breathing is meditating. You can also buy cds to help guide you in your meditation, if you are not sure about what you have to do.

- There are herbal teas or even hot milk which people have used to help them to relax.

So make sure that you get enough sleep so that you have the energy to tackle each day at your best.

Step 12—Shop well

When you go shopping it is so easy to reach for that packet of chocolate biscuits or that "economy" sized packet of chips. Fast track to when you are at home in the evening watching TV, what do you reach for besides the remote control? That is right; you end up snacking on that packet of chips or chocolate. If you are prone to eat out of boredom, having these foods in your cupboard will only tempt you to eat them.

Next time you go shopping, buy the healthy snacks such as fruit, low fat snacks such as rice crackers, dried fruit and nuts. As I said earlier there are no bad foods, so if you really do need that chocolate buy a small bar rather than the 250 gram block. I know they have the snack sized chocolate bars where there are 15 portions in one packet. However, this will only make you eat more. So just buy a few portions of what you would like.

You will find that once you have said your affirmations that you will just not feel like eating certain types of foods. It may be hard to believe as you sit there on your first night watching TV and wondering why you just did not buy that extra packet of chips. However over time you will not even remember that you have that packet of chips sitting in the cupboard. Or you will know the chips are there but just will not want to eat the chips.

Step 13—Eating disorders

When you think about your body, weight and food most of the time, and you use harmful methods such as starving yourself, vomiting and diuretics to lose weight, you have an eating disorder. There are hospital programs which show women and girls how to eat properly so that they can recover from their illness. That is they need to eat regularly every couple of hours and they need to eat food such as fresh vegetables, fruit and meat. This is important and if you have an eating disorder you need to get some professional help.

A bit of background about your past can help your counsellor give you the appropriate treatment for you. A lot of how we feel about ourselves relates to what has happened to us. Many women may have been either emotionally or physically or sexually abused. You may have been brought up in a way so that you do not discuss your problems with people outside the family. Some women with eating disorders do not even realise that the real problem is more psychological. Their eating disorder may in fact be a coping mechanism to deal with what has happened in their past or is happening to them now. Eating disorders are complex and each case should be treated separately.

To recover from your eating disorder you need to open up to a trusted counsellor. Do not feel embarrassed or ashamed as they are trained to deal with women and girls who suffer with an eating disorder. The professional will give you a diet plan and then also work with you to deal with your other issues in another way. You need to let go of the people and the circumstances that made you feel bad. Once you have let go of the people and circumstances which made you feel bad, you can then start learning to love yourself, your body and your spirit.

The previous chapters helped you identify ways of making you feel better about yourself. Surrounding yourself with people who treat you with respect is also another lesson that women or girls who suffer from eating disorders need to realise. If anyone in your life makes you feel scared or unworthy, then you need to change that relationship. There is assistance in the way of counsellors and even anonymous help lines. You have to believe that you are fantastic and that you are great just the way you are.

Sasha's story

Sasha grew up in a household where there was domestic violence and she lived in fear for most of her life. Her parents fought constantly and she always felt as though she was walking on egg shells.

During her childhood her parents were constantly criticizing her and would tell her that she was 'fat'. Sasha started to believe the words that she heard and believed that she was naturally overweight. She suffered from an eating disorder for years and never made the connection between her family and the eating disorder. When she was 18 her parents became so concerned about her eating disorder that they took her to see a doctor. Sasha joined a hospital program where she had to record everything she ate. She had to ensure that she had three main meals and three snacks throughout the day. Sasha would visit the hospital one afternoon a week and submit her diet sheet.

However Sasha found that she was unable to get along with her parents so she moved out of home. She continued to see her doctor and after a few months, her eating disorder disappeared. During this period Sasha had ceased all contact with her parents. She started feeling good about herself and relieved that she was able to overcome her eating disorder.

One year later Sasha's mum contacted her and wanted to see her again. Sasha agreed to see her parents again and after a few months she moved back in with her parents. A couple of weeks after living with her parents, Sasha's eating disorder started again. She felt like a failure and was ashamed of her behaviour. She was back in the control of her eating disorder, and the next five years were a struggle with both Sasha's parents and her illness. Then one day she had a particularly bad argument with her parents and she moved to another town.

Once she was in the new area and had reduced the contact with her parents, Sasha recovered from her eating disorder. She stopped dieting and found that her life started to be peaceful. The eating disorder was a coping mechanism for Sasha as her parents behaviour made her feel bad about herself. Since she had known them all her life, she never realised how they had affected her.

Eating disorders are sometimes mechanisms for you to cope with the emotional pain you are suffering in your life. You need to work through the pain with a trusted counsellor and distance yourself from relationships which hurt you emotionally. Words can sometimes resonate longer and more deeply than any physical pain. Unlike a physical blow, words do not leave a scar. So you cannot see the damage to your mind and spirit. You need to be treated with respect and kindness. No one should ever make you feel dreadful no matter what you have or have not done. People who make you feel bad do not have your good intentions at heart. Unfortunately sometimes close family members are the ones who make you feel bad and you have to stand up for yourself and your happiness.

Step 14—What happens when you are at your perfect weight?

When you have lost weight and reached your goal weight, what thoughts run through your mind? Do you rejoice at losing weight but have a niggling feeling that you will put the kilos back on? I have heard of so many people who have lost weight but they keep their old clothes just in case you regain it? What is that saying to yourself? You are telling yourself that you are going to put the weight back on, so you better keep your old clothes.

When you have reached your goal weight, get rid of all your old clothes that are too big for you, I mean all of them. Give it to charity as there are always people who will need clothes. You have lost the weight and it is not coming back, so you do not need your old clothes which are now too big. Believe that you are naturally slim and so you do not even have to think about losing weight. Use the affirmations and the visualisations every day to make you believe that you are naturally slim. Whenever you feel bad about your body from now on swap the thought with an affirmation. Always see yourself as naturally slim in your mind and believe that you are.

Step 15—What do you do now that you are naturally slim

Most of you would have spent so much energy thinking about your weight and body image, that you did not have enough time to do or think about anything else. Forget about your weight and start doing all the things that you want to do now.

Is there an interest or a hobby that you have always wanted to do? You now have that time, so go and start doing your hobby. Is there a book that you have always wanted to read? What about travelling or going on a holiday? Did you want to learn to sew, paint, or draw? You now have the time to do whatever you want, so go out there and learn.

A lot of you may feel a little lost as you do not know what to do with your free time. I suggest that you try different things until you find something that you enjoy. Some suggestions are:

- Start to look at how you can understand money
- Go to the library and borrow some books to read
- Help out your favourite charity
- The library is also a great place to research other things that you enjoy
- Learn how to scuba dive
- Learn how to ride a horse

- Plan your holidays and be adventurous
- Follow your dreams

Life is great and you can now enjoy it, as you will no longer be worrying about your weight. I have shown you all the steps to be the naturally slim body you were born to be. So go out there and enjoy your life and forget about trying to lose weight. There is a whole world out there waiting for you to explore it.

Chapter 4

Money

Changing your relationship with Money

Developing your financial ability gives you more choices and freedom in your life.

Your financial ability has to be developed similarly to how a baby starts to walk. You all first started by crawling, you then carefully took your first steps, walked around, and then once you were comfortable with walking, you started to run. Developing your financial ability is just the same. You need to crawl first before you can walk and then run. The important thing is to make sure that even when you stumble over, you still get up and keep trying again. So never give up trying to understand money. This book will help you with your baby steps so that you gain the confidence to understand finances and eventually take control of your life.

Our understanding of money is important to all of us because it gives us control of our own lives. You cannot rely on others to look after you financially. In my life, I have met many women in unhappy situations because they thought that money was too difficult to understand. All these women were worried about money and felt trapped in their situations. The reality is that they still have the power to make changes so that they can be happier. They just need to gain confidence in relation to managing money so that they can take control of it and live comfortably and peacefully.

I will first show you the steps you need to follow to start managing your money. Towards the end of this chapter, you will then be given real life examples of women who have applied the steps, and now manage their own finances and their own lives. Do not worry if you do not fully understand each step of what you have to do, as the scenarios towards the end of this chapter will give you real life examples. You may find that you need to read the chapter more than once and then go back and follow the steps. The main goal is for you to gain the confidence in understanding and managing your money. This is not a race so take your time and open your mind to understanding money.

Step 1—Finding the motivation

The first step on the road to financial freedom is to find YOUR reason for wanting to be financially independent. My reason for being financially independent is so that I can make the decisions in my life and look after my children. I have always wanted a balanced lifestyle so that I could work, spend time with my family and have time to pursue my interests in writing and art. My overall reason for wanting to be financially independent is so that I can live my life the way I want.

Everyone is very different and you need to find your own reason for wanting to understand money. This part is up to you and here are some ideas of why you need to be financially independent:

1) For yourself—gives you independence and more choices in your life.
2) Your retirement—for many of you this may be a long way off. However this depends on when you plan to retire. Society's concept is that you work and work while you are young and save your money and build up your assets. Then when you get to sixty, you stop working and then start to relax and enjoy your life. Does that idea sound good to you? Let us look at it in another way. Maybe you could set yourself up financially at a much younger age, so that

you have more time to enjoy your life and do the things that you enjoy. How does the idea of retiring at forty sound to you?

3) Your Family—More time with your family as you can afford to work part time or not at all. Children grow up very quickly and before you know it, they have moved out and are leading their own lives. It would be great to be able to be around your children as they are growing and needing some direction and guidance from you.

4) People get divorced and even if your marriage does last, what are you going to do if you outlive your partner and your partner has been the one to manage the finances.

5) Your children—You can support your children and give them what they need such as a good education and take them on life changing holidays.

6) Charities or causes you would like to help. Do you love animals and would love to be able to donate time or money to help an animal shelter?

7) Doing the things that make you happy such as travelling. Imagine yourself walking the streets of Paris or even lying on a beach sipping on a cocktail.

8) Other reasons—Sit down and make a list of what you want now and in the long term and what makes you happy.

Once you have found your own reason or reasons, write it down. You will notice that your reasons will have very little to do with money. Saying you want more money will not give you more money. So every time you feel as though you are losing interest in understanding money, look at the reason that you have written down. This reason has to be something that makes you happy to get up every morning and motivate you to understand money.

Step 2—Finding the time

Too many of us make excuses about why we cannot find the time to do something. Do you remember when you really loved doing something and you somehow found the time to fit it in? When we have a family, work, study or do all three, our days are full. If we are mums with young children, we will be looking after them all day and then collapse into bed each night. Even if our kids are school age, there is the morning rush as we get the kids ready for school, and then do our housework or run errands while they are at school. Then pick them up after school, feed them, help them with their homework, get them to have their showers and then get them to bed. Most mums are literally exhausted at the end of each day.

You may not have kids but work full time. When work has finished for the day, you might go to the gym or do some other activity. By the time you get home you are tired and mentally and physically drained. So most of you have a pretty packed day and you try and fit in as much as you can.

When you find your own reason about why you want to be financially independent, then that reason will motivate you to find the time to keep learning about money and not give up.

I want to be able to look after my kids as they are very important to me. So that motivates me to spend an hour each night, either reading books, watching dvds or even checking the internet about money.

Step 3—Setting Goals

Write down your goals for 3 months, 6 months, I year, 2 years, 5 years and even 10 years. You can choose whatever time period you want and you do not have to do all the time periods. Make the goals specific and give them a deadline that is relevant to you. Think about what you want or where you want to be in the future. The goal has to make you feel good when you achieve it. If you are not confident about your finances, then your first goal may be:

E.g. 3 months—I will understand my finances and have read one financial magazine, article or book by 30 September 20XX.

Choose a goal that you are comfortable with and one that you would like to achieve. It is very important to be specific about your goals, and put down the time frames. This will allow you to focus more on what you want

Step 4—Love what you do

In order for you to earn money you need to love what you do. This may be a job or your own business. First of all decide what you would like to do and then look at how you would go about getting into it. Check out the internet (libraries have free access to the Net) and once you get some ideas of possible training courses, start ringing around to see how you can get into it. Where there is a will, there is a way!! It is amazing how the doors will open for you once you have decided what you want to do.

I have held different jobs during my life time. In order to do well, I had to feel passionate about it. What I liked changed over time, so I would then try another position. You can even have more than one job. For instance, I have my day time job where I love working with numbers and at night I love writing.

My comfort level lies in working for an employer and investing in property. Others prefer to own a business. Everyone is different and you have to be able to sleep at night. The key is to decide what you love to do and then go for it. You will be amazed at how everything will flow, once you have decided what path you want to follow.

Step 5—Mind set

This might sound strange but changing your mind set is an essential part of your financial education. You need to change the way you think about money. If you do not have the right mind set, you will not be able to learn about finances and have money in your life. One of the reasons that many people who win lottery lose all their money within a few years is because they do not have the right financial mind set.

You have to believe that you deserve to be financially independent and that you deserve to have money in your lifestyle. You may have grown up in a household where money was seen in a negative light. For instance, that people who want to be rich are greedy. Money is not bad, nor is the desire to have it. Money allows you to make choices which can help you and your family to lead a comfortable lifestyle. It also allows you to help out your favourite charities and help your community.

Your self-esteem may be low and so you subconsciously believe that you do not deserve to have money. Sit back and look at how you feel when you have money. Do you feel uncomfortable about having it? What thoughts come to your mind, when you think about money? Are they good words or bad words? How do you feel about having a lot of money in your life? You may want to have more money in your life. However, if you associate negative words with money or if you feel that you do not deserve to have it, then money will not enter your life.

Clarinda's Story

Clarinda was a divorced mother of two children. She always felt 'empty' and did not believe that she was 'good enough'. This applied to all areas of her life including relationships with men and money. Clarinda was always struggling with money and always seemed to be in debt. She never realised that as long as she felt bad about herself as a person, money was never going to enter her life. Subconsciously Clarinda is telling herself that she is not worthy of having it. Whenever she gets any extra money she spends it on 'stuff' for her and the kids. So while she may be saying she wants more money in her life, she keeps spending it whenever she gets it because deep down inside she feels that she does not deserve to have it.

Look deep within yourself and how you think about money. Do you use it to make you happy and then feel guilty for spending it? Remember that you are a great and smart person who deserves to have money in your life. It is about living in the now and allowing yourself to have money now. Your money habits in the past are exactly that, in the past.

It is never too late to change your beliefs so decide today that you are going to make changes now. Today is the beginning of the rest of YOUR life with money. So starting today allow yourself to have it in your life.

Your goal is to have the mindset of a wealthy person who feels good about money. How do you think wealthy people feel about money? Do they worry about it? Do they wonder if they have enough money to pay the bills every day? The answer is no. Wealthy people have a very different attitude and feeling towards money. They never worry about having enough of it. In fact they feel good about money and their main focus is on how to make more. Wealthy people have a positive attitude towards money and they have a "wealthy" mind set. You have to change your attitude towards money and adopt a positive mindset about it.

Step 6—Affirmations or mantras

Saying daily affirmations will help you to change your mind set about money, so that you can start feeling good and positive about it. Affirmations or mantras are phrases that when said repeatedly will help change the way you think. As you go through your day, listen to what your thoughts say about money. If you are having money problems then chances are that your thoughts are full of negative comments about not having enough of it. Affirmations will help you change your thoughts so that they are more positive. You will be amazed at how different your life will be once you have started to include affirmations in your life. Affirmations need to be said as many times as you can a day. Whenever you have a negative thought about money, then swap it straightaway with a positive thought such as "I have plenty of money". If you do this whenever you have a negative thought about money, you will then see that your finances will get better as you are now confident about having more in your life. You will also start to feel very differently as you stop worrying about money.

Examples of affirmations are:

I am good at managing money.
I am open to receiving money from all sources.
I have plenty of money.
I deserve to have money in my life.

Another helpful way to help change your attitude towards money is to have affirmations written on pieces of paper and posted around your house. So that whenever you look at the pieces of paper you have positive words to say. You can make up your own affirmation about money. At the end of the day, the affirmation has to be believable for you!!

Step 7—Be inspired by the success of others

What are your thoughts when you hear that someone is successful and is wealthy? Do you get jealous? When you get jealous, you are blocking any money from coming to you, as you think that the other person has money, so there is not enough money for you. The reality is that there is enough money for everyone, including you. So the next time you hear that someone is wealthy, use it as inspiration for yourself. We are all able to have plenty of money in our lives and we should use successful people as inspirations for ourselves to succeed. So next time you hear how Olivia Johnson bought a house . . . think . . . If she can do it then I can too!

Step 8—Everyone can be smart with money

My grandmother told my mum, who told me, that a woman should always be financially independent. She should have her own job so that she can be independent and earn her own income. My grandmother was born before World War 2, but she had the foresight even then to realise the importance of financial independence. My mother passed on this advice to me and my sisters. I followed this advice and discovered that in addition to earning your own income, you should also invest your money.

I studied accounting at university; however those studies did not provide me with skills to manage my own money. I know accountants who live in debt because they are unable to manage their personal finances. My financial ability was gained through reading lots of books and asking lots of questions. You never stop learning and I continue to read and learn every day.

We are not all born with an instant financial ability. Men do not know more than women, or vice versa.

We are all equal when it comes to the ability of being financially savvy. The key is to believe that you can understand money. These are some of the steps in educating yourself financially.

- You—you are the best person to manage your money. You trust yourself and you know that you will make decisions to look after number one, which is you. Too many people think managing their money means getting their financial advisor or accountant to manage their money. Financial advisors and accountants have their place. However at the end of the day, you need to know exactly what money you are receiving and where you are spending or investing your money.
- Read books—libraries are a great way to find the books that suit you. Remember there are thousands of books out there about money, so you need to keep borrowing or buying books until you find one that you can relate to.
- Internet—there is plenty of information on the internet about understanding finances. Remember however that this is about understanding money. So do not go "shopping" for someone else to manage your finances or buy products that you do not really need. This is an information gathering exercise only and does not cost you anything.

- Government or charitable organisations—it is now recognised that women need to develop their financial abilities and there are programs available from governments and charitable organisations. There are services run by organisations that provide information to women on their finances.
- Attend free courses and seminars
- Speak to friends and family about how they manage their money. You would be amazed at what ideas you can learn from simply speaking to other people. Do not ask them about how much they earn, it is more about asking how they manage their day to day finances. Just listen and see what they say. You then use your own judgement and decide if you want to follow some of their advice. It can also be a way of seeing what you should not do!

Everyone can be smart with money and it does not have to cost you anything to educate yourself.

Step 9—Making money

Good Debt and Bad Debt

Good debt is debt that you have created from your investments, while bad debt is debt related to "stuff" like clothes and shoes that you have bought.

In this age of credit, young people are finding themselves in credit card debt even before they have their first full time job. It is so easy to go to a bank and get a credit card. They now have them in various colours so you can choose one in your favourite colour!! *Credit cards can be used but need to be fully paid off every month.* So when you get your monthly statement you need to be able to pay the full amount owing on the statement, not the minimum repayment. The last thing you want to do is to owe money on your credit card after the minimum payment date, and have to pay interest on this amount. A better alternative is a debit card, where you use your own money. You never pay any interest as you are using your own money.

How do you get out of bad debt?

If you find yourself in bad debt, then this is one way of getting out of it.

1. Firstly, take your credit card out of your wallet and leave it at home. This will stop you from buying things on the spur of the moment that you do not need.
2. Then set up an automatic payment system to pay off your bad debt and forget about it. Yes you heard right, you need to forget about your debt and think about making money. For

instance, have $50 a week that is automatically taken out of your savings account to pay off your credit card. Just set up the repayment and forget about your debt. The more you focus on debt, the worse you will feel and you will want to spend money to make yourself feel better. This will only create more debt. So forget about it.

3. If you have a number of credit cards with varying amounts of debt, then get one personal loan to repay all your credit card debts. This is also called "consolidating" your debt. So instead of having three credit cards totalling $3,000, you will have one personal loan totalling $3,000. Then set up an automatic direct payment system between your loan and savings account and forget about your debt. Always try to pay more than your minimum payment if possible. You then have to cancel two of the credit cards, leaving only one. Reduce the limit of your last credit card and keep it at home. Utility bills like electricity and gas can be paid using a credit card, however day to day purchases such as clothes or groceries should be paid with cash.

4. Starting today, change the way you use a credit card. You only need one to pay for regular bills and leave it at home. When you do use the credit card, make sure that you pay it all off by the minimum payment due date. You

do not pay the minimum repayment amount only by the due date, as this will increase your debt over time. So make sure you have the money in your savings account to pay off your credit card in full, by the credit card minimum payment due date.

5. After you have set up the automatic payments, start to focus on setting up a budget or money maker (explained later) and creating wealth. Dwelling on your past debt, will only create more debt in your future. You have to believe that you are financially fine now and trust that your automatic payments will repay your debt.

It can be hard to stop focusing on your debt when you keep receiving bills in the mail. So you need to find a way to pay your bills automatically and not think about them. When you receive your bills, check that it is right and then just pay them. Do not worry about future bills as they have not arrived as yet. We all have to pay for various things in order to live. Another way to help you change your mind set about bills may be to think that the company who sent it to you, trusts you to pay for their services. You are lucky that they sent it to you. Find a way to change your attitude towards bills in a more positive way.

Many people put the bills on the fridge or somewhere where you look at them all the time.

This will only make you think more about debt. Put the bills in a place where you do not have to look at them every day. A suggestion may be to have a filing system where once a week you look at all the bills that are due in that week and then pay them. Most people have mobile phones today, so you could record reminders in your phone to pay your bills. Find a system that will help you pay the bills without having to look at them every day.

Put something positive on the fridge such as a strategy to help you make money. Even an article about wealth will help you think about making money rather worrying about debt. Your main goal is to pay your debts off by an automatic payment system and focus on making money.

Step 10—Do you really need it?

This next section may be a bit confronting but you need to hear this, if you want to have money in your life. You only buy things that you really need. For instance you have a party to go to and instead of wearing an outfit that you already have, you decide to go out and buy a new outfit. There are special occasions where you do need a new outfit but most of the time, there is at least one outfit that your friends have not seen you in. You are not celebrities who will be photographed by the media and need to make sure you are not wearing the same outfit twice. You can also buy skirts, tops and pants, so that you can change the look of your outfit by mixing and matching different clothing.

There are also many of you who buy your children 'stuff' that they do not need. Your children need love, food, clothing, shelter, education, and your time. Buying your children stuff every time you go out, is only teaching them bad habits about spending. This is also teaching them that you need stuff to be happy. Look at your spending habits and what you spend your money on. Do you really need everything that you buy for you and your children? What would happen if you did not have it? In your honest opinion, would your children get more out of spending time with you or a toy that they would lose interest in within an hour? Spend money on experiences for yourself and your family.

I have met many women who claim that they are worried about their credit card bill but will continue to buy things with money that they do not have. The best way to avoid this from happening is to leave your credit card at home, as this will stop you from impulse buying. The second thing you can do is to only go to the shopping centre when you have to buy something specific. Window shopping is the main reason that you end up buying things that you do not need. If you have issues with your credit card, just walking around in a shopping centre will cause you to spend money that you do not have. So instead of going shopping, go for a walk outside, watch DVDs, read a book, talk to your family or visit a friend. There are plenty of things to do in life rather than just shop because you are bored.

It is also important to say your affirmations daily as this will create a mindset that will allow you, to make the decisions to bring money into your life. So instead of feeling as though you are depriving yourself from shopping, you will discover a whole other life not involving spending money. This will actually make you and your family happier.

Step 11—Managing your money and only spending what you have

After my divorce, it took me a while to get into the right mindset. I had always been very good at managing my money. However, after my divorce I found that I had lost my confidence. My spending habits were out of control and I was actually indulging in . . . wait for it . . . "retail therapy". You know, that is when you go and buy 'stuff' to make you feel better. My retail therapy was disguised under necessity, as I was buying groceries as though I was waiting for a cyclone to hit. Only trouble with that is that your happiness is short lived once you see the credit card bill. (Note—I always fully paid off my credit card statement each month so that I did not pay interest). I then read about changing your mind set using affirmations, so I started saying them every day.

After saying my affirmations and changing my mindset, I then set up a budget or money maker. I do not know about you but I do not like the word budget. The word makes me feel as though I am being punished, as I cannot spend as much as I want to. So I called my budget "Karen's Money Maker". The name made me feel as though I was making money rather than depriving myself of it. You can name your budget anything you want but the underlying message is that the budget will give you the lifestyle choice you want in the long run. In order for the budget to work properly, you have to work out your income and expenses, and this will enable you to only spend the money you have.

Reason you do not have enough money in your life

The reason that you do not have enough money is because you spend more than what you earn. Even if you did earn more money, chances are you would still spend more money than what you earn. This is the main reason why so many people who win lotto, end up losing it all after a few years. They do not know how to manage their money by using a budget. *A budget will ensure that you only spend the money you have.*

Money maker or budget

I will now call a budget a 'money maker' so that you will have a positive attitude towards using a budget to manage your money. The money maker will help you stay on track, so that you only spend the money you have. The first step is to see how much money you receive and then what you are spending your money on. This will show you exactly how much money you have left each month after paying all your bills. The next step is to then see what changes you can make, so that you can have more money in your life.

The first step in developing your money maker, is to see what you are spending your money on now.

Income

Income is money that YOU RECEIVE now. It is money from your job, business, the government, interest from savings etc. Each source of income is listed separately according to how much money is received each month. Look at payslips, letters and bank statements if you are not sure.

Expenses

Expenses are what you spend in order to live. For instance, your rent, mortgage, groceries, electricity, water, rates, mobile phone etc. Do not look at bills as something negative or bad. Everyone has bills and you need it in order to live. So the next time you get your electricity bill, just accept it and be grateful that you have electricity. There are many countries that do not have this basic need.

To help you work out your expenses go through your credit card statements and past bills. Think of EVERYTHING that you would spend money on. Another tactic to help work out how much you spend is to collect all the receipts for the past fortnight. When you do this exercise, you actually see how much you spend and on what you spend it on. I am warning you that this is not for the faint hearted. You would be amazed at how much you spend on little things. Every transaction can add up to a significant amount.

Money left over—surplus or deficit

Once you have collected information on what you spend your money on, you will see exactly where your money is going. This is where you need your basic maths skills of addition and subtraction. You need to look at all your income and expenses for the week. Take away your expenses from your income and the difference is either your surplus or deficit.

Income minus expenses equals what you have left over

Income—expenses = Money left over (surplus) or money you do not have (deficit)

Surplus is when you have money left over from your income after paying for all your expenses. This is great as it shows that you are only spending the money that you do have.

Deficit is when your expenses are more than your income. So that means you are basically spending money that you do not have. All this means is that you have to look at doing things differently, so that you only spend the money that you do have.

Whatever your position is, there are a number of things that you can do to help bring more money into your life. First, start by looking at each expense and deciding if it is a need or a want. A need is what you need to live (food, rent, electricity, and water) and a want (kids toys, jewellery, Friday night drinks, eating out) is something that you would like to have but can live without. Then look at whether you can reduce the expense.

The following are examples of expenses that you can look at to bring more money into your life.

Rent—This is a need and can be reduced by finding a cheaper home or someone to share with.

Mortgage—This is a need and you can look at reducing your repayments by shopping around at different financial institutions to get a cheaper interest rate. Sometimes your own financial institution may give you a better deal if you just simply ask them. Remember to check for any hidden costs if you make any changes to your mortgage. You can also make fortnightly repayments rather than monthly repayments. This will stop you from spending the money on things you do not need. Another way to help you with your mortgage is to get someone to share with you. This will help reduce your mortgage payments, as well as your other bills such as electricity, water etc.

Groceries—This is a need and can be reduced by a few ways. Here are some suggestions on reducing your grocery bill:

- You can have a shopping list and stick to it when you go shopping.
- Only go shopping by yourself so that you only spend money that you want to. This may help all those mums who find that their children will nag them to buy more items.
- Make sure you are not hungry when you go shopping, as this is when you tend to buy more than what you really need.
- Choosing home brands for generic products such as sugar, flour, toilet paper etc.
- I found that the best way to control your spending on groceries is to pay for them using cash. For instance you would allocate $150 for groceries, so each week you would take out $150 cash from the bank. You would pay for your groceries using the cash you have. This ensured you would stick to your budget.
- I found that when you use your credit card to pay for groceries, you did not know how much you actually paid for groceries, until you received your credit card statement.
- Another tactic is to keep all the receipts you spend on groceries each week. Once again this will help you stick to your money maker.

These are only suggestions and you may know a better way of reducing your grocery spending.

Mobile Phone, home phone, internet—There are plenty of service providers around and you can look around for a cheaper option.

Utilities such as your electricity, water and gas—Many service providers will allow you to pay them regularly so that by the time you get your bill, you have actually paid most of it. For instance you can agree to pay $30 each fortnight to your electricity provider when you first connect it. So by the time you get your first bill, in 2 months' time, you have already paid for most of it and in some cases the whole bill. This is a great way to make sure that you only spend the money that you have.

Stuff—As mentioned earlier do you really need all the stuff that you buy? When I first started working I met a lady who told me that she spent over $100 on gossip magazines each month. That was amazing as she eventually admitted that she was always "broke". Is there something that you are spending money on now that you do not really need?

The main idea is to go through all your expenses and see what you can do differently so that you can reduce your expenses. Once you have set up your money maker and start to follow it, you will see that you will have plenty of money in your life and you are on your road to having a more positive attitude towards money.

Step 12—Charity is another important category

When you start to feel comfortable with money, you will also need to start donating part of your income to charities. Donating to charities will make you feel good, as you realise that you are actually helping others. When you do give to charity, you have to give from your heart. You will find that the more you give to charities, the more money you will receive. Money needs to flow and helping out charities allows money to flow into your life, as well as the lives of others. I have always donated to charities and find it personally rewarding. Donating to charities makes you feel as though you have plenty for yourself and that you are able to give to others. It is also changing your mind set to the belief that you have plenty of money. Do not donate if you feel uncomfortable about giving. Donating needs to make you feel good so only donate to a charity you believe in, when you are ready to give happily.

Step 13—Saving money is essential and you will need to save a certain percentage of your income

Saving money is essential to help you plan for your future. It helps you buy something that is more expensive than what you have allocated for your weekly spending. For instance, you would like to buy a dress for a party and it costs $200. Instead of using your credit card to pay for the dress, save a little each pay day until you have your $200 to buy your dress with cash. You will feel a sense of achievement and you will appreciate your dress more as well. More importantly you will not have debt sitting on your credit card, long after your party is over.

A part of your income needs to be deposited in a savings account, each time you receive money. Make sure you cannot take the money out of this account easily, so that you are not tempted to spend it when you are out shopping.

When you have a savings account, you can then buy the things you need straight away without having any debt. Start by saving a small amount each week, say 10% of your salary or earnings in an account you do not have ready access to. Build this up; say 10% to 20% to 25% to 30%, until you are saving 30% of your salary or earnings in a savings account. It may take you a while to build it up but eventually 30%

of your salary should be going towards your saving's account. This allows you to buy something that you need or invest the money. Many women do not have their own savings account. I have even heard of a case where a woman's savings account was in her husband's name only.

Susie's Story

Susie had a savings account where she deposited part of her salary each month into her husband's Pete's savings account. Whenever she needed money she had to ask him for it. Susie and Pete eventually divorced and Pete refused to give Susie any money from this account or allow her to take any furniture from their home. Susie was left in an emotional and financial mess.

This is not the way to set up a savings account. If your partner refuses to have a joint savings account (i.e. both your names are on the account and you both can take money out), then you need to set up your own savings account in your name. It is a good idea to have your own savings account where you deposit a small amount regularly. Even $20 every two weeks will eventually add up. You need to know that you are able to look after yourself financially should anything happen.

Step 14—Investing

Once you increase your money through your savings account, you also need to grow your money, by investing it. The word may sound complicated but all it means is to increase the money you earned from your job or business. I chose to invest in property as I was interested in it. However, you may find that some other type of investment suits you better.

Choose an investment that interests you, so that you find it an interesting or fun activity. If it feels like too much hard work, there is a danger that you will lose interest and not do well. Here are some ways of helping you decide on the type of investment that suits you best:

- Read books—libraries have books available on various types of investments. There are also motivational type books which will help you to stay on track with your investing and your future.
- Subscribe and read magazines which specialise in investments—there are many magazines that will help you invest and they explain it in easy to understand language. So next time you are at the news agents, skip the gossip magazines and head straight for the money and investment type magazines.

- Attend courses and seminars—There are free information sessions held by community type organisations or government organisations. So ring them up and see what is on offer in your area.
- Speak to people who have already done it. Before I bought my first ever investment property, I met a work colleague who had investments. I asked him about what he did and how he did it. I found he was quite happy to talk about it and share his knowledge. He eventually became my first mentor.

Golden Rule

The golden rule is that whatever type of investment you choose you have to be able to sleep well at night. There is no point in following someone else's advice blindly and then finding you are stressed and anxious. Everyone has a gut instinct and women are lucky, as you have women's intuition. Trust your gut instinct and walk away if you feel pressured or unsure about any advice that you receive. Do not worry that you will upset the other person. You have to look after yourself and your family and if your gut instinct is saying that something is not right, then walk away.

Here are more tips on investing:

1. Do your research.

   When I first started, I read books by various property investment authors, and I asked different investors questions about investing, until I was able to decide how I wanted to approach property investing. Months of research preceded me buying my first property.

2. Only speak to people who have successfully invested.

   There are plenty of people out there who are more than happy to find reasons about why you should not do something. So make sure that you only discuss investing with people who have successfully invested in the areas that you are interested in.

   When I started investing, there were many people who had never invested in property, who would tell me about all the bad things that could happen. These are people who have never done it. Do you want to be like them? If you are serious about investing, look around and get advice from people who have been there and done it successfully.

3. Start small.

When trying out anything for the first time, it is best to start small. So if you are interested in investing in property for instance, buy one first and see how the process worked. What strategies worked for you? What strategies could you improve? Once you have worked out your strategies, then go on and purchase more properties. The same goes for any type of investment.

4. Once you feel confident move up a step.

That first step is always the hardest. Investing may be out of your comfort zone and the whole concept may sound too complicated. However, once you see that you can do it the first time, it gives you the confidence to keep creating more investments.

5. Get a mentor.

It is hard doing anything by yourself. You would be surprised how people are willing to help you for free if you just ask them. In order to succeed it helps to have someone who has already done it. I am not talking about getting someone to do everything for you. I am talking about having someone you can bounce ideas off. Be careful here though. Like everything else make sure that before you make any final decisions, you follow your gut instinct. If they suggest something that does not sit well with you, then do not follow their advice. They are there to only guide you. I have had several mentors over my life in relation to investment properties. Each one suited me for the stage I was at. I did not follow their advice blindly, as I always did my own research and calculated my own figures.

6. No such thing as failure

Remember there is no such thing as failure, only lessons to be learnt. There have been many successful people who have suffered disappointments before they reached their goal. When something does not go as planned, do not beat yourself up and think that you are a failure and that all those negative people were right. You have to take a step back and look at what you have learnt from your experience. Then try again and use your experience to succeed the next time. Each experience brings you one step closer to your goals.

Step 15—Overcome your fears

Fear is the number one factor that stops people from doing anything with money. What if I lose it all? What if I cannot make my repayments? What if I lose my job? What if I lose my house? What if the world ends? What if? What if?

Most of us have these thoughts, I know I did. However, you have to push past these thoughts. You have to be optimistic and take baby steps to ensure that you succeed. Use your affirmations to replace any negative self-talk.

I always believe that things work out for my best interest. When I was looking to purchase my investment properties I believed in my heart that I was going to buy a good investment. I only spoke to people who were positive about property investment, ignoring people who were pessimistic and who were all too happy to tell you why it was not good to invest in property. If you look at those negative people's lives you will see that they have probably never looked at investing but are quite happy to bring you down.

Finally—Real life examples

Applying the strategies to real life women

To help you apply the strategies that I have just discussed, I will show you how some of the women I have met, have successfully applied the strategies. When I first met them they had allowed others to take control of their finances, and they were unhappy. They then applied the strategies and are now managing their own money and their own lives. I have modified the money maker figures in the examples to help you understand the figures more easily.

Lisa's Story

Lisa is a thirty two year old, smart, and vibrant woman with two children aged three and five. She found the courage to leave her husband after an unhappy marriage. However, after 6 months on her own, she found her financial situation tough. Lisa gave up working after having children and now relies on government benefits, and child support from her ex-husband, John.

When Lisa was married, John earned enough money so that she never had to work. Lisa did not worry about money and would buy whatever she wanted, as there was always money in the account. However, now that Lisa was separated, she found herself having problems with money. After a few unexpectedly high bills, Lisa plunged into debt and tried to survive day to day. The more she tried to get out of debt, the more her debt grew. John also became more difficult. The man whom she had fallen in love with, had turned into a cold stranger who begrudged paying her any money. Lisa could not believe that life could be so stressful and even contemplated returning to John just so she could fix her money problems.

Step 1—Finding the motivation

Lisa was sick of having sleepless nights and worrying about money. She wanted to be able to have enough money to look after her children and herself.

Step 2—Finding the time

Lisa decided to spend three nights a week reading about money and working through her finances. She went to the library and borrowed some books about money, then read them once the kids had gone to bed.

Step 3—Goals

Lisa started by jotting down her short term and long term goals.

3 month goal—Have a part time job with greater hours so there is a balance between working and spending time with her children by 31 Aug 20XX.

1 year goal—Lisa wants to be a nurse, so she started applying for courses. Lisa hopes to get into her course by 31st December 20XX.

3 year goal—complete her Nursing course and start working which will give her more money and stability by December 20XX.

4 year goal—own her own house by 31 May 20XX.

Step 4—Love what you do

Lisa had wanted to be a nurse since she was a little girl. However she had met her husband when she was seventeen and he did not want her to study at university. So she had married relatively young and had never managed to start the nursing course. Lisa now decided that she would start her career as a nurse. She applied for a nursing course in several institutions, sat for the entrance test and after a few months was told that she was successful in gaining entry into two universities. Lisa started her course and was amazed at how happy and positive she was starting to feel about her future. She could see that she and her children were going to be alright after all.

Step 5—Mind set

Lisa grew up in an abusive household. Her parents fought constantly and she was subjected to physical and emotional abuse herself. Not surprisingly, Lisa grew up with very low self-esteem, and deep down she felt as though she was not good enough. When Lisa looked at how she felt about money, she realised that she never felt as though she deserved it. Lisa had to look deep inside herself to finally realise that this was her attitude towards money. She had also spent money to make herself feel better.

In order for Lisa to start having more money in her life, she needs to realise that she deserves to have it. She has to start allowing herself to have more money and to feel good about herself and work on herself esteem.

Step 6—Affirmations

Lisa started to say affirmations every day. She stuck them around her house so that she would think about them all the time. Whenever she felt bad about money, she would swap the thought with a positive affirmation. Her attitude towards money started to change as time went on and became more positive. Here are some of her affirmations.

I deserve to have money in my life
I have plenty of money
I am good at managing money
I allow myself to have money in my life

Step 7—Be inspired by the success of others

Lisa did not know anyone personally whom she thought was successful until she started her nursing course. She met other older women who had also decided to study nursing and before long, she had a group of friends who were all helping each other and inspiring one another to do well in their course and succeed in life.

Step 8—Everyone can be smart with money

After working on understanding money Lisa realised that anyone could be great with it. Her daily affirmations were working and she was slowly changing her attitude towards money.

Step 9—Making money

When I first met Lisa she had credit card debt and was having sleepless nights. Lisa made the effort to stop using her credit card and to pay for everything with cash. She paid off her credit card through weekly automatic repayments and is now saving her money.

Step 10—Do you really need it?

Lisa's biggest weakness was buying stuff for her kids. Whenever she went out, her children would "nag" her for toys and anything else that they saw. Lisa toughened up and started to say no to her children, more often, without any explanation as to why they could not have it. Lisa would just say "NO" and after a few weeks, they reduced the amount of times they asked for things. Lisa had grown strong enough now to say no without feeling guilty.

Step 11—Money maker

In order to show you how Lisa's money maker was developed I will remind you of her background when I first met her and then the changes she made to take control of her finances.

Lisa is a single parent who has two children and is studying to be a nurse. Lisa had no idea about finances and was never taught how to spend her money. She grew up listening to her parents saying that they did not have enough money and then watched them as they spent money that they did not have. The irony is that while Lisa could see what her parents were doing in relation to money, Lisa never realised that she was doing exactly the same thing. Every day Lisa got up feeling overwhelmed by her bills including her credit card bill.

Lisa received $1,000 a fortnight from government benefits and she received $200 a fortnight from her ex-husband for child support. So in a fortnight she has an income of $1,200. Lisa also kept all her receipts for a fortnight to find out exactly what she spent.

Before		
Fortnightly (2 weeks) Income		
Government Benefits	$	1,000
Child support	$	200
	$	1,200
Rent susidised	$	400
Water	$	20
Electricty	$	30
Phone/Internet	$	75
Gas	$	20
Mobile	$	30
Groceries	$	300
Entertainment/toys	$	350
Credit Card Repayments	$	253
Total Expenses	$	1,478
Money Left Over	-$	278
Credit Card debt $5,000		

Her receipts during the two weeks showed Lisa that she had spent $350 on buying toys and other 'stuff' for her family. These are items that she did not really need but bought while she was at the shopping centre. She was also paying too much for her home phone and internet.

When Lisa looked at the numbers, she realised that she was spending more than she was receiving. Lisa decided to stop using her credit card and started paying cash for everything. Paying cash makes Lisa realise just how much money she is spending. Handing over a credit card to pay for $100 worth of groceries, is a different feeling from paying with cash. When Lisa pays with cash, the reality of exactly how much she is spending hits home.

Lisa also decided to reduce her credit card debt by using an automatic payment from her savings account to her credit card. Looking at all the bills and receipts, Lisa looked at what she could do to reduce her bills. She decided to shop around and eventually found a cheaper home phone and internet provider.

After a year and a half Lisa had paid off her credit card debt and was now able to save money.

After		
Fortnightly (2 weeks) Income		
Government Benefits	$	1,000
child support	$	200
	$	1,200
Rent subsidised	$	400
Water	$	20
Electricity	$	30
Phone/ Internet	$	50
Gas	$	20
Mobile	$	30
Groceries	$	300
Entertainment	$	100
Credit Card Repayment		
Savings	$	100
Total Expenses	$	1,050
Money left over which Lisa can put in her savings account	$	150
Or pay her credit card		
Credit Card debt is Nil and is fully paid off each month		

Lisa now has more money in her life and all she had to do was make a few changes in her money maker.

Step 13—Charity is another important category

When Lisa was feeling more confident with her money, she started to donate to some children charities. She loves children and wanted to help others that were in more difficult circumstances. Lisa found the act of giving very fulfilling as she was helping to make a difference.

Step 14—Savings

Lisa paid off her credit card and is now saving money so that she can eventually have a deposit for a home for her and her children.

Step 15—Investing

At this stage Lisa is still researching various types of investments and is talking to different people about the many options. She plans to start investing after she has purchased a home.

Step 16—Overcome your fears

Lisa's greatest fear was getting into debt and losing everything. She had to push past her comfort zone and make the effort to understand money. As time went on she realised that money was not as difficult as she had always believed.

Where is Lisa now

Lisa is a nurse and is now enjoying working at a hospital. Her children are happy as they can see that Lisa is no longer stressed. Her new career and her understanding of finances have increased her self-esteem so that she is positive about her family's future. Lisa is now in the process of buying her own home and her life is getting better. When she looks back, she is amazed at how far she has come in her life. The unhappy, stressed single parent is now a confident and successful woman.

Maria's story

Maria had been married to Robert for over 20 years. On the surface it appears that they have a great relationship, as Maria is a teacher and Robert is a successful Executive. They have two beautiful children who are away at University. Maria and Robert own a beautiful home and drive the latest cars. Both Maria and Robert enjoy a very comfortable lifestyle of holidaying overseas, fine dining and designer clothes. However, Maria is hiding a horrible secret. She learnt that Robert was having an affair after reading some text messages on his mobile phone. When Maria confronted Robert, he denied it but the text messages on his phone were far from businesslike and he continued to have his late night meetings. Maria was unhappy in her marriage and she wanted to leave Robert. However, Robert controlled their finances and earned the most money. If Maria left Robert, she was not sure if she would get the money she was entitled to, as she had left the "money side" to Robert from the moment they had married. Maria knew they had money but she did not know where all the money or investments were. She also did not know how much money she and Robert actually had. Since Maria was nearing retirement, she was not sure if she had enough money to support herself during her retirement if she left Robert. So Maria stayed in the marriage out of the fear of not having enough money, to live the lifestyle she had grown accustomed to.

Step 1—Maria's motivation

Maria wanted to learn about money so that she could make decisions about her retirement and future. She wanted to be able to leave Robert if he was unwilling to work on their marriage. She wanted to gain the confidence to ask Robert to go to counselling and see if they could save their marriage and needed to know that she would be able to lead her own life and be financially secure, if her marriage ended.

Step 2—Maria finding time

Maria decided that every night she would devote one hour of her time to understanding money.

Step 3—Maria's goals

Maria sat down and wrote out her goals.

3 month goal—understand her and Robert's personal finances by 31 August 20XX

6 month goal—work on her marriage by going to a marriage counsellor by November 20XX

1 year goal—change in career to increase her income by 30 June 20XX

5 year goal—retire and work part time by 1 January 20XX.

Step 4—What Maria loves to do

Maria loved teaching and she wanted to make a difference in more children's lives. When she started teaching she had been busy looking after her family as well as working. Her children were now older and they did not need her around anymore. So Maria decided to look at Deputy Principal roles, where she would have more interaction with parents and children. She also started to join committees and take courses to help her gain a role as a Deputy Principal. The new role would also give her more income. Maria started to apply for Deputy Principal roles and after a year, was successful in gaining a Deputy Principal role at another school. Maria was surprised at how her new role made her feel confident about herself. It also made her realise that once she put her mind to it, she could achieve whatever she wanted.

Step 5—Changing Maria's mindset

Maria had grown up in a traditional household where her father had controlled the finances. It seemed only natural to let her own husband Robert look after the money side once they got married. Maria had a joint account with Robert. He paid the bills and would tell Maria how much she could spend. Maria had to realise that she could look after her own money. So she had a talk to Robert and told him that she wanted to share in the responsibility of their finances. To her surprise, Robert did not argue against the idea. Maria opened up her own bank account and redirected her salary to her new account. She then started to sit with Robert each night to learn exactly what money, bills and investments they did have. Each step Maria took was liberating and made her feel like a stronger person.

Step 6—Maria's Affirmation

Maria used the affirmations below and started saying them every day. She felt too uncomfortable to have her affirmations around her house, so she kept her affirmations in a journal, which she would look at each morning and each night before she went to bed. At work her computer password was always something positive about money. When she got a bit worried about money she would swap the thought with something positive about money.

I am smart and I am good at managing money.
I deserve to have money in my life.
I am respected and loved.

Step 7—Be inspired by the success of others

When Maria looked at her friends, she realised that a lot of them actually took an active role in managing their family's finances. One friend in particular named Tasha, ran her own business and was financially successfully. In the past Maria had felt slightly envious of her friend's success and was bored by her conversations about business. However, now Maria looks at her friend Tasha for inspiration, and discusses ideas about making money. She is now motivated by Tasha's success and realises that if Tasha could do it, then she can do it too.

Step 8—Everyone can be smart with money

Maria realised that anyone can be smart with money (Maria was an English teacher). She began to see that just because she was not good at maths in school, did not mean that she would be bad at managing money. After sitting with Robert each night, to learn about their finances, Maria realised that he was pretty clueless about money. Robert also had credit cards which with large limits. He did not follow any type of system and was basically spending more than they both earned. Maria was surprised that Robert really did not know what he was doing after all. She also found out that Robert had purchased an apartment that was making a significant loss. A lot of their money was going towards the investment loan repayments. Robert explained to Maria that he had never mentioned any of their finances to her in the past, as he thought that she was not interested. After listening to Robert explain his ideas about their money, she realised that understanding money was not as difficult as she had always believed. Maria started feeling better about money and both she and Robert started managing their finances as partners.

Step 9—Making money

Maria and Robert had a few credit cards that she had used unthinkingly. They were paying interest on all of them and had only ever paid the minimum balance by the monthly due dates. Maria now destroyed all but one of her cards. To reduce her debt, she set up an automatic payment between her savings account and her credit card. The repayments were more than the minimum payments for each card.

Step 10—Do you really need it?

When Maria looked at her spending habits, she realised that her Saturday ritual involved her going shopping for clothes and shoes. She did not need the clothes but shopping just made her feel better; it filled the emptiness she felt. Maria started to change her Saturday routine and no longer shops every Saturday. She has started to do other things like going for walks, catching up with friends or spending the time reading. Maria still occasionally shops for clothes and shoes, but only because she needs it.

Step 11—Money maker

Maria had found out that Robert was not following a money maker so she sat down with him one night and together they worked out their money maker based on what they were currently spending.

Before	
Monthly Income	
Robert's Salary	$ 12,500
Maria's Salary	$ 5,000
	$ 17,500
Mortgage	$ 3,500
Water	$ 50
Electricity	$ 50
Phone/ Internet	$ 200
Gas	$ 50
Mobile	$ 200
Groceries	$ 2,400
Entertainment	$ 350
Credit Card Repayments	$ 998
Investment Property	$ 4,000
Savings	$ 3,500
Charity	$ 3,500
Total Expenses	$ 18,798
Spending money than what they have	-$1,298
Credit Card Debt $20,000	

Maria realised that they were losing money every month from their investment property. In co-operation with Robert, they sold their investment property and purchased another one, which gave them back more money. They started paying extra on their credit cards and also used their savings to reduce their credit card debt. They are now saving more money and are planning to use their savings on a family holiday.

Their new money maker now looks like this:

After	
Monthly Income	
Robert's Salary	$ 12,500
Maria's Salary	$ 5,000
Investment property -rent left after paying all expenses	$ 100
	$ 17,600
Mortgage	$ 3,500
Water	$ 50
Electricity	$ 50
Phone/ Internet	$ 200
Gas	$ 50
Mobile	$ 200
Groceries	$ 2,400
Entertainment	$ 350
Savings	$ 3,500
Charity	$ 3,500
Total Expenses	$ 13,800
Money left over each month	**$ 3,800**
Credit Card debt is Nil and is fully paid each month.	

Step 13—Charity is another important category

To Maria's surprise Robert had already been donating to a number of charities, which made Maria regain some of her respect for him, as she had never truly appreciated how generous he really was.

Step 14—Savings

Robert had a "savings" account set up but Maria did not have access to it. Maria went to the bank with Robert and created a new savings account, with joint access.

Step 15—Investing

As mentioned earlier, Robert had invested in an apartment that was making a loss. That is, the rent from the property did not cover the loan and other property expenses. After reading some books, and doing research, Maria and Robert decided that they needed to sell the apartment. They eventually sold it and bought another property that was positively geared. This means that every month the rent they received from the apartment paid for the loan on the apartment as well as all the other property expenses.

Step 16—Overcome your fears

Maria had always been worried that she would make mistakes and lose everything. However, now that she is actually making an effort in managing her finances, she is gaining more confidence and her fears are slowly disappearing. The more she reads and researches, the more her confidence grows. Maria realised that putting her head in the sand previously was actually worse as she knew nothing about her own money. It led her into a situation where she felt trapped and powerless in her own marriage. Maria now realises that she has nothing to lose and everything to gain by understanding money.

Where Maria is now

Maria eventually gained an understanding about managing her finances and learned about all the investments that both Robert and she had. She had also started to create her own investments in shares. This gave her the confidence to discuss the marriage problems that she and Robert had in their marriage and they decided to go to counselling. Maria was no longer feeling trapped and she and Robert were still together. She was now an equal partner in the marriage and she was no longer worried about suddenly being single and broke.

Maria's understanding of finances has given her the confidence to think positively about her future and her retirement.

Cassie's Story

Cassie is a 25 year old successful sales person who works in real estate. She is single, lives in an exclusive part of the City, always wears the latest in fashion, drives an expensive car and projects herself with a wealthy facade. The reality is that she is broke and is in significant credit card debt. Cassie knows that she is in debt but she cannot seem to get out of it no matter how hard she tries. Like Lisa, the more she tries to get out of debt, the more her debt grows.

Step 1—Finding the motivation

Cassie wants to take control of her money and her life.

Step 2—Finding the time

Lisa has decided to spend half an hour each night learning about money.

Step 3—Goals

3 month Goal—Follow her money maker and learn about money.

1 year Goal—Follow her money maker and save 10% of her salary.

2 Year Goal—Buy her own apartment by 31 May 2015

3 Year Goal—Travel to Europe by 30 June 2016

Step 4—Love what you do

Cassie loved her job in the real estate agency she was employed at so she continued working in her role there. However she decided to get fitter by going for a walk each morning. This helped to clear her head and get her in a positive mind set for the start of each day.

Step 5—Mind set

Cassie had a great childhood and her parents gave her everything she wanted while she was growing up. However she had learnt her spending habits and mind set about money from her parents. They had always bought whatever they needed on credit card and were always in debt. Cassie had grown up listening to her parents talking about 'stuff' that they wanted to buy and putting everything on the credit card. They also talked about increasing their credit limit whenever they reached their credit limit. Cassie realised that she needed to change her mind set towards credit if she wanted to get out of debt.

Step 6—Affirmations

Cassie had never been good at maths in school so she had always believed that she was not good with numbers. Since money involved numbers, she had believed that she would also be bad with money. Cassie is now saying her affirmations daily and her confidence in managing money is getting better.

I have plenty of money
I am good at managing my money
I deserve to have money in my life

Step 7—Be inspired by the success of others

Cassie works in the real estate industry and is surrounded by people who are property investors and talk about making money all the time. In the past she has found their conversations about investing intimidating. She never thought that she would ever have enough money to invest however she can now see that it is possible to save money. Cassie is interested when someone mentions anything to do with investing or money. She has learnt a great deal simply by listening and asking questions.

Step 8—Everyone can be smart with money

Cassie is now realising that anyone can understand money. Reading about it each night is helping her to understand her money and making her feel confident about managing her own finances.

Step 9—Making Money

Cassie had $40,000 credit card debt which was made up of 4 credit cards. She had to get a personal loan for $40,000 and pay them all off. She then cancelled three of her credit cards and reduced the limit of the last credit card to $2,000. She then set up an automatic payment system so that $500 a week was going towards paying off her personal loan. Cassie had to set up a money maker so that she could make extra payments and reduce her loan more quickly. She then left the credit card at home and started to plan for her future.

Step 10—Do you really need it?

Cassie's biggest weakness was clothes, shoes and Friday night drinks after work. All three left a huge dent in her purse. She started to look at her lifestyle and made an effort to stop spending money on things that she did not really need.

Step 11—Money maker

When Cassie first gathered all the information about her income and expenses, she realised that she was spending more than what she earned.

Before	
Monthly Income	
Cassie's Salary	$4,615.00
Total Income	**$4,615.00**
Rent	$2,167.00
Water	$ 50.00
Electricity	$ 50.00
Phone/Internet	$ 200.00
Gas	$ 50.00
Mobile	$ 200.00
Groceries	$ 400.00
Entertainment	$ 350.00
Credit Card Repayments	$1,992.00
Savings	
Charity	
Total Expenses	**$5,459.00**
Spending more money than what Cassie has	-$ 844.00
Credit Card Debt $40,000	

She then paid off her credit card and ensured that every month she paid it off in full. Cassie still goes out and buys clothes, but she has reduced the amount she is spending on her stuff. She moved to an apartment which was a lot cheaper than her previous home and after changing her spending habits, she is now making more money.

After	
Monthly Income	
Cassie's Salary	$4,615.00
Income fron property investment	$ 100.00
Total Income	**$4,715.00**
Rent	$1,517.00
Water	$ 50.00
Electricity	$ 50.00
Phone/Internet	$ 200.00
Gas	$ 50.00
Mobile	$ 200.00
Groceries	$ 400.00
Entertainment	$ 300.00
Credit Card Repayments	$ -
Savings	$1,385.00
Charity	$ 100.00
Total Expenses	**$4,252.00**
Saving Money	**$ 463.00**
Credit Card Debt is Nil and is fully paid for each month	

Step 13—Charity

Cassie had never donated to any cause previously so she did some research. She loved animals so she decided to donate to a charity that helped them.

Step 14—Savings

Cassie started to save some of her salary and now that she had cut down on her shoes, clothes and Friday night drinks, she is finding it easier to save money.

Step 15—Investing

Cassie is now investing in property as she has met a co-worker who has agreed to be her mentor and give her direction. She is amazed at how easy investing is and wishes she had started earlier.

Step 16—Overcome your fears

Cassie's biggest fear was living in debt forever and losing everything. However now that she has made the changes in her life, she is reassured that there will be plenty of money for her future.

What is Cassie up to now

Cassie is now the happiest she has ever been. She is no longer in debt and she has started to invest in property. It amazes Cassie that in the past she had always shown investors properties. However she had never thought about investing for herself, as she was always feeling as though she did not have enough money. She has now purchased her own apartment and is working on securing another investment property for herself. Cassie is enjoying her new found freedom and appreciates the fact that she can go through her day without worrying about money.

Summary of changing your relationships with Money

Remember—Developing your financial ability gives you more choices and freedom in your life.

Step 1—Finding the motivation—Decide why you want to understand your finances.

Step 2—Finding the time—Make time to learn about your finances. Your reason will keep you motivated to find the time.

Step 3—Goals—Set goals about where you want to be in your future.

Step 4—Love what you do—Work or start a business in an area that you are interested in.

Step 5—Mind set—Be aware of your attitude towards money and make an effort to have a positive attitude starting today.

Step 6—Affirmations—Create affirmations and have them placed throughout your home so that you can start to change your mind set about money and believe that you are good at managing it.

Step 7—Be inspired by the success of others—When you get jealous of someone else's success, it blocks money from entering your life. Next time you hear that someone is wealthy, use it as an inspiration for you to succeed in your life. If they can do it, then I can too.

Step 8—Everyone can be smart with money. You just need to educate yourself by reading books, magazines, watching dvds or even attending seminars.

Step 9—Making money—Debts should be paid using an automatic payment between your savings account and your debt. Then forget about your debt and focus on making money.

Step 10—Do you really need it?—Look at your purchases and decide if you really need it. Avoid impulse buying by making a shopping list.

Step 11—Money maker—the money maker or budget helps you to only spend the money that you have. This will help keep you on track so that you can save and eventually invest for your future.

Step 13—Charity—donating to causes that are close to your heart will help money flow into your life and also change your mindset, so that you have a positive attitude towards money.

Step 14—Savings—save a percentage of your salary so that you can purchase more expensive items and also invest the money for your future.

Step 15—Investing—investing your money allows you to increase your money so that you have a more secure future. However always ensure that you do your research thoroughly before investing any money. Also listen to your gut instinct before investing any of your money, as you need to be able to sleep at night when you make your decisions. Remember there is no such thing as failure, only lessons to be learnt.

Step 16—Overcome your fears—a lot of people do not do anything about money because they are fearful. Only speak to people who are positive about money and are successful. This will keep you focused on succeeding in your goals.

The final word

You have been provided with the strategies to take control of the finances in your life. A basic money maker or budget will help you save money and eventually invest it. This is the "technical" part of understanding money and the only part involving numbers. The rest in relation to understanding money has very little to do with numbers. It has to do with you and what you want in your life. It is important that you say your affirmations about money daily, so that you can change your mindset and start to really believe that you are good at managing money. Place those affirmations around your home, so that you see them wherever you go. The most important thing is to never give up on yourself and your own ability to understand money. There is plenty of money for everyone, so make the decision today that you want to understand your finances.

So I sincerely wish you all the best in developing this new skill as everyone can do it and I know YOU can!!

Chapter 5

Key Strategies

At the end of the day, your happiness is in your hands. You are the only one who can change your life. Many of you keep saying that you will be happy when you get that new job, that new house or even that man you have dreamt about. Unfortunately you will find that having extra stuff or a partner does not make you happy in the long term. In order to feel better about life you need to work on yourself first. Do the things that will make you feel good about you as a person.

It is totally up to you if you want to make positive changes in your life. Too many people read a book and miss the message. This is because the person is not ready to make any real changes in their life. You will not magically feel better just because you read the book. Be honest with yourself and look at your life to see what changes you can make to have a better life. The strategies that have been suggested have to be put into place by you. YOU need to want to make the changes for yourself. Perhaps you need to read this book more than once to find out what will work for you.

Another way to look at life on this planet is to see that your time on earth is similar to being in a classroom. That is, you are faced with different experiences both good and bad. Each event teaches you something about yourself and others. Since we are all individuals with our own personalities, only we can work out what we have learnt. So when you are faced with a difficult time, take a step back and try and see what lessons you can learn. It may be that you realise how strong you actually are.

While I was finalising the writing of this book, my work underwent a restructure and I was suddenly faced with the prospect of being unemployed. I was understandably upset by the circumstances and had sleepless nights as I lay awake and thought about my future. My whole work area was depressed as everyone was going through the prospect of losing their jobs. When you go through such an event, it can bring out the best and the worst in people. I met some great people during this period whom I would never have normally met.

To improve my chances of finding other employment, I decided to retrain and gain some new skills. So I approached our training area and asked the team if they could organise some basic training for me and some of my work colleagues. The training area did not have to agree to the training, as they normally trained a different section of our organisation. However they were empathetic to my circumstances and agreed to conduct the training. Prior to this, the trainers had only been names on an email list, as I organised the payment of their utilities. However due to the restructure, I met these people face to face and suddenly my whole perception of them changed. They stopped being names on an email list and became people who were generous in spirit. I saw another side of them. They were also facing the loss of their jobs but were happy to help me and my work mates out. If it was not for the restructure, I would never have met these people and seen how kind they could be.

In summary here are the key strategies that have been discussed:

Relationships

- The most important relationship is the one you have with yourself.
- Your issues with your weight and money relate to how you feel about yourself.

- If you feel bad about yourself then you are going to have issues with your relationships, weight and money.
- Be kind to yourself and realise that you deserve to have the best in life.
- You are a good person and you deserve to be happy.
- Do things that will make you feel good about yourself.
- Look at the people who are currently in your life and whether they make you happy.
- Always trust your gut instinct about people.
- If you have negative unhappy people around you then chances are you are also slightly negative.
- You can change this part of your personality so that you are more positive about life and yourself.
- Change any negative relationships by letting people know how you feel. This will give them the chance to change the way they treat you. If however they continue to treat you badly then you may have to see less of them.
- The rule to follow is that the people in your life are meant to make you feel good most of the time.
- Any relationship can have its ups and downs, but if you feel low whenever you spend time with a person. Then you need to decide how

you are going to change that relationship for the better.

- If you are scared of a person then you definitely need to let them go. No one should feel scared of someone in their life.
- Repeat everyday "I **have positive and loving relationships in my life.**"
- Replace any negative thoughts about relationships during the day with your positive affirmation.
- Sometimes there are people in your life who try to make it difficult. There is nothing you can do to change them. The only thing you can control is your attitude towards them. My suggestion is to bless them and send them love whenever you think about them. This will help you focus on the positive.

Lose Weight

- In order to lose weight, first focus on making yourself feel better on the inside.
- This is where you need to work on the relationship you have with yourself.
- Rule out any other issues which may be causing you to be over weight. Some women subconsciously put on weight so that they can protect themselves. So take a hard look at

yourself and see if you are overweight because of an issue.

- If there are any issues, get the help of a good counsellor who can help you work through your problems.
- Then use affirmations to change your mindset, so that you believe you are naturally slim. When you get up each morning you believe that you are naturally slim and there is no need to lose weight.
- Start thinking like a slim person, affirm every day that **"I am slim and healthy."**
- Use visualisation so that you see yourself as slim in your mind's eye. So that whenever you think of yourself, you see the slim person that you are.
- Exercise every day to make yourself feel better. Allow yourself to eat anything you want, so there is no "bad food" and any temptations in your life. Allow yourself a few pieces of chocolate, if that is what you want. If you deny yourself certain foods like chocolate, then chances are that you will end up eating a whole block of chocolate later.
- Instead of focusing on losing weight, focus on being your ideal weight.
- So if you want to be 70 kilos then say "I am 70 kilos" whenever you think about your weight.

- Replace any bad thoughts about weight you may have during the day with your positive affirmation.
- You will be amazed at how free you will suddenly feel once you have forgotten about losing weight.
- Life is meant to be about different experiences not staring at yourself in the mirror every day, reading the scales and feeling miserable.
- Start to focus on your life today and let go of any thoughts about losing weight.

<u>Making Money</u>

- As mentioned earlier, you need to feel good about yourself on the inside so that you can start having more money in your life.
- The key to making money is to change your mind set to believe you deserve to have plenty of money.
- Work on your self-esteem so that you feel good about yourself.
- It is also important to spend less money than what you earn.
- You will need to set up a budget (or money maker) and stick to it.
- Leave your credit cards at home if you know you are the type of person who cannot control your spending.

- Credit cards need to be paid off in full on the minimum payment due date, instead of only paying the minimum amount.
- Expensive items should be purchased from the money you saved, instead of using your credit card.
- Debt is to be paid off by automatic repayment so that you can focus on making money.
- Do NOT focus on your debt as it will only lead to a vicious cycle of more debt.
- Do focus your energy on sticking to your budget or money maker and saving money to invest.
- Most importantly, trust your gut instinct about people and investments. Use what you have learnt about money and investing to work out if your fear is real or just fear of the unknown.
- You need to affirm every day that "**I am good at managing money and I have plenty of money. I deserve to have money in my life.**"
- Swap any bad thoughts about money with your positive affirmation.

What I have learnt so far in life:

- My family are a blessing and have taught me about unconditional love.
- My health is important, and I am grateful for being alive every morning.

- I am responsible for my own happiness.
- I treat others the way I want to be treated, that is with respect, compassion and kindness.
- I have to let go of the past as I cannot change it no matter how much I think about it.
- I do focus on what is going on in my life now.
- Sometimes things happen in my life, which are out of my control. However I decide how I react to the situation.
- Having dreams and goals is essential in making me happy and giving me a purpose in life.
- Buying things such as a bigger house, nicer car will only make me happy for a moment and not bring me true happiness.
- One of the happiest times in my life was a beautiful day at the beach with my family.
- While money cannot buy happiness, I need balance in all areas of my life, including finances.
- Helping others and giving from the heart makes me feel good.
- I accept my body and there is no need to diet.
- The people around me reflect how I feel about myself.
- There is plenty for everyone and I am happy to share.

Your Life

During your life time you will have many experiences. The main idea that you need to realise is that you have more control over your life than you think. You are the one who decides how life is going to turn out, no one else. Sometimes things happen to you which are out of your control; however your reaction to the experience is within your control. You can be bitter and angry or you can let it go and move on with your life. Hanging onto bad experiences will only make you feel bad and it will eventually affect your health. Realise that you deserve to feel good, so after feeling angry for a set period of time you choose, you need to let your bad past experiences go.

In circumstance such as someone you know dying, it is ok to be sad and grieve. Sad is different from being depressed and negative. Allow yourself to grieve for a period of time then you need to let the sadness go and move on with your life.

As the old saying goes, birds of a feather flock together. This means that you will attract people who are like you in their mindset. When you have a more positive mindset, you attract more positive people and experiences. If you are unhappy and depressed, then chances are you are going to have people in your life who are going to make you unhappy. So open your eyes and look at the friends and family you have in your life now.

A lot of people think that their life will improve once all their 'problems' are resolved. Change your mind set to believe that your life is good now and feel happy, then your life will be happier. So do not wait for tomorrow to be happy or for that new house or car. Start today and enjoy your life now.

Make an effort every day to be positive no matter what is happening in your life and to think of affirmations that will make you feel happy. Live your life to the fullest and realise that life does not have to be hard; it can be a joyful experience. The most important message I would like to pass on is to believe in yourself and your ability to attract and maintain supportive relationships, be your perfect weight and have plenty of money in your life.

Karen's quick and easy-to-follow guide is for the busy woman who wants more positive relationships, weight loss, and more money. She received her wakeup call when she found herself at the lowest point of her life during her divorce. Everything in Karen's life seemed to be in a mess, namely her relationships, weight, and money. Karen thought that surely life was not meant to be so difficult. So she started to search for some answers to her questions such as:

- Why do I attract the same type of relationships?
- How do I attract positive relationships?
- How do I lose weight and keep it off?
- How can I have more money and support my children?
- How can I live the type of lifestyle I want to lead?
- How can I be HAPPIER?

Karen read a variety of books, and each author helped her to fine tune her life-changing strategies. She found out through personal trial and error what worked and what did not work to improve her relationships, weight, and money.

When Karen looked around, she saw that many of her friends had to deal with similar issues. In fact, many women were struggling to deal with their relationships, weight, and money. Karen started to help other women and found the experience was extremely rewarding. So she then decided to write this book so she could draw from her own experience to help more people. Karen details the strategies she has learnt to help lead a happier life. She knows how busy women are, so she has written an easy, step-by-step guidebook which will show you the strategies to make positive changes in your life.

ভঃ

Karen is a busy mother, accountant, property investor, coach, and writer who loves walking and reading. She is a motivational coach who has a passion to help people believe in themselves so they can have more positive relationships, achieve weight loss, and have a better understanding of money.

AU $23.99

ISBN 978-1-4525-0936-5

9 781452 509365

BALBOA
PRESS

A DIVISION OF HAY HOUSE

Los Molinos
The Windmills

...and other Selected Translated Poetry of Juan Parra del Riego

Selections of Juan Parra del Riego:
Chosen, Edited, and Translated by Dr. Dennis L. Siluk Ed. D.
Three Time Poet Laureate (& Rosa Peñaloza de Siluk)

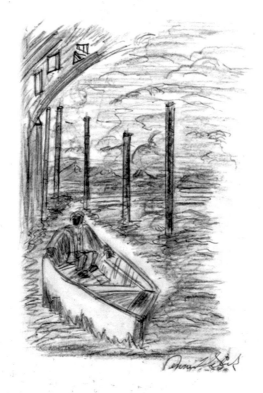

"This book is going to be a bestseller!"
Apolinario Mayta, Journalist Editor for the *'Primicia,'*
Newspaper for Huancayo, Peru

The Council (ruling body) of the Continental University of
Huancayo, Peru, congratulates and recognizes

Dr. Dennis L. Siluk, Ed.D.